Evolution in Dental Care

Evolution in Dental Care

Edited by

Richard J. Elderton BDS, PhD

Professor of Preventive and Restorative Dentistry
Department of Conservative Dentistry
University of Bristol
UK

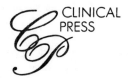

CLINICAL
PRESS

Published by Clinical Press Limited,
Redland Green Farm, Redland Green, Redland, Bristol, BS6 6HF

British Library Cataloguing in Publication Data

Evolution in dental care
1. Dental services
I. Elderton, Richard J.

362.1'976

ISBN: 1-85457-020-X

Lasertypeset by Martin Lister Publishing Services, Carnforth, Lancs

Printed in the UK by Antony Rowe Ltd, Chippenham, England

Contents

List of Contributors

(*invited contributor to the conference)

Y.E.Y. Aboush, Lecturer, Department of Conservative Dentistry, University of Bristol, UK

A.K. Adatia, (formerly) Professor of Dental Science and Clinical Practice, University of the West Indies, Jamaica

K.J. Anusavice*, Professor and Chairman, Department of Dental Biomaterials, University of Florida, Gainsville, USA

D.E. Barmes*, Chief, Oral Health, World Health Organization, Geneva, Switzerland

D.K. Benn, Research Fellow, Joint Department of Community Dental Health and Dental Practice, University College and Middlesex School of Medicine, University of London, UK

R. Bornstein (and **M. Zimmerman, T. Martinsson**), Department of Oral Diagnosis, Karolinska Institute, Huddinge, Sweden

E.M. Bronkhorst (and **W.J. Kluter, A.J.M. Plasschaert, G.J. Truin**), Department of Cariology and Endodontology, with **M.F.H.G. Wimmers**, Department of Social Gerontology, Faculty of Psychology, University of Nijmegen, and **J.H.G. Klabbers**, Department of Gamma-Informatica, University of Utrecht, The Netherlands

W.P. Crocker, General Dental Practitioner, Buckingham, UK

T.W. Cutress*, Director, Dental Unit, MRC of NZ, PO Box 27007, Wellington, New Zealand

E.S. Davenport, Lecturer (and **J.M. Hardie, J.M. Smith**), Department of Child Dental Health, The London Hospital Medical College, UK

T.B. Dowell*, Regional Dental Officer, South Western Regional Health Authority, Bristol, UK

M.C. Downer*, Chief Dental Officer, Department of Health, London, UK

A.J. Drinnan*, Professor and Chairman, Department of Oral Medicine, State University of New York at Buffalo, USA

R.J. Elderton*, Professor of Preventive and Restorative Dentistry, University of Bristol, UK

L.V. Foster, Lecturer, Department of Conservative Dentistry, University of Bristol, UK

M. Gazi, Assistant Professor (and **A. Moran**), Division of Periodontics, College of Dentistry, King Saud University, Ryadh, Saudi Arabia

E.R. Gordon, General Dental Practitioner, Hendon, UK

C. Hall Dexter*, Dental Practitioner, London, UK

M.H. Hobdell*, Professor, Department of Community Dental Health, Preventive Dentistry and General Practice, University of Dublin, Ireland

C.J. Holmgren, Lecturer, Department of Periodontology and Public Health, University of Hong Kong

S.M. Hooper, Lecturer, Department of Conservative Dentistry, University of Bristol, UK

G.F. Howden, Senior Lecturer, Department of Conservative Dentistry, University of Hong Kong

N.W. Johnson*, Nuffield Research Professor of Dental Sciences, Department of Dental Sciences, Royal College of Surgeons of England and Honorary Director, MRC Dental Research Unit, London Hospital Medical College, UK

B. Ksiazkiewicz-Jozwiak, Department of Prosthetic Dentistry, Medical Academy of Cracow, Poland

E.M. Kuzmina*, Assistant Professor, Moscow Medical Stomatological Unit, USSR

B.S. Lembariti*, Senior Lecturer in Periodontology, University of Dar es Salaam, Tanzania

K.L. Lester*, Professor of Dentistry, Westmead Hospital Dental Clinical School, Australia

A.P.A. Luukkonen, Consultant, MMC Dental School Development Project, University of Kuopio, Finland

M.L. MacIntyre, Preventive Dentistry Co-ordinator, Saudi Aramco Oil Company, Dhahran, Kingdom of Saudi Arabia

L.C. Martens, Assistant Chairman, Department of Conservative Dentistry, Pedodontics and Preventive Dentistry, University Hospital, Gent, Belgium

M. Midda, Head of Periodontology, Department of Oral Medicine, Surgery and Pathology, University of Bristol, UK

P. Nitisiri*, Director, Intercountry Centre for Oral Health, Chiang Mai, Thailand

S.L. Perera, Senior Lecturer, School for Dental Therapists, Columbo, Sri Lanka

T. Pilot*, Professor, Faculty of Dentistry, University of Groningen, The Netherlands

J.J. Pindborg*, Professor of Oral Pathology, The Royal Dental College, Copenhagen, Denmark

V.G. Pinto*, National Oral Health Director, Ministry of Health, Brasilia, Brazil

N.B. Pitts, Director, Dental Health Services Research Unit, University of Dundee, Scotland

J. Sardo Infirri*, Scientist, Oral Health, World Health Organization, Geneva, Switzerland

C. Scully*, Professor, Department of Oral Medicine, Surgery and Pathology, University of Bristol, UK

W.C. Shaw*, Professor of Orthodontics and Dentofacial Development, Department of Oral Health and Development, University of Manchester, UK

A. Sheiham*, Professor of Community Dental Health and Dental Practice, Joint Department of Community Dental Health and Dental Practice, University College and Middlesex School of Medicine and the London Hospital Medical College, University of London, UK

B.P. Singh, Head, Department of Dental Surgery (*and* **I.C. Tiwari**, Professor of Community Medicine), Institute of Medical Sciences, Banaras Hindu University, Varanasi, India

C.D. Stephens*, Professor of Child Dental Health, University of Bristol, UK

H. Tala*, Assistant Chief Dental Officer, National Board of Health, Helsinki, Finland

A. Tewari*, Professor of Pedodontics and Preventive Dentistry (*and* **K. Gauba**, **V. Sachdev**, Assistant Professors; **K. Ashima**, Senior Research Officer; **N. Kaur**, Senior Resident), Postgraduate Institute of Medical Education and Research, Chandigarh, India

F.K. Wahab, Research Assistant, Department of Conservative Dentistry, University of Bristol (*and* **R.P. Shellis**, Senior Scientist, MRC Dental Group, Bristol Dental School), UK

S Warnakulasuriya, Professor of Oral Medicine (*and* **A. Ekanayake**, Professor of Community Dental Health), Peradeniya, Sri Lanka

T.F. Watson, Lecturer, Department of Conservative Dentistry, University College and Middlesex School of Medicine; Research Fellow, Department of Anatomy and Developmental Biology, University College, London, UK

Preface

This is a book for all those involved in dental care, especially those who wish to participate in decision-making that will advance the speciality and thereby shape tomorrow's dentistry. It is also for those who will be affected by the way dental care is evolving at present. The prospect of an improved quality of life is assuming an increasing importance in many different parts of the world. High-quality health care is central to this aspiration. Within general medicine, the hope of more and better dental care is especially prominent because dental and oral diseases are so common and widespread. In the face of this demand, many countries and indeed many individuals need to commit themselves to important decisions that will markedly affect the oral health of their peoples and patients for decades to come.

The world is an ever-changing place and change in dentistry is occurring very rapidly indeed. In countries where restorative treatment has dominated the scene, many shortcomings have become apparent. These have added impetus to the beginnings of a move towards developing much more of a preventive philosophy. Also, scientific knowledge of the common dental diseases is advancing rapidly, and the effects of new diseases are exerting a major influence upon the way dental care is carried out – prevention is thereby taking on a new meaning. Another major change is that levels of dental caries have fallen dramatically in most developed countries during the last 10 to 15 years, while in many parts of the developing world the levels are rising fast as social structures change and diet patterns are modified in response to economic development.

The concept that individuals, wherever they may live, can be wholly reliant upon organized dental services for the maintenance of their oral health and function is fast becoming an illusion as our understanding increases and as the true costs become apparent. All dental practitioners need to know what is over the horizon so that they can attune their practices for optimal relevance in the future – patients move with the times and dentists need to be one step ahead. Thus, serious questions have to be asked, now, about the treatment-orientated dental practice that is still prevalent in the UK and in other industrialized parts of the world.

Can and should dental caries and other oral diseases be managed largely by preventive means? What forward-looking decisions should dentists be making, whether they are practising within a highly treatment-based structure or if they are working in a developing area? Will the developing countries follow in the footsteps of the 'Western world' with traditional restorative dentistry, or will more and more of them aim directly for prevention so that restorative dentistry is deflected from becoming the main thrust of their future oral health services? Will it be that the 'Western world' eventually falls into line with a preventive approach pioneered in developing areas?

These and many other issues were discussed at the international conference *Decisions in Forward-looking Oral Health Care* held at the University of Bristol on 7–9 September 1988; and it is the deliberations of this conference that form the basis of this book. The familiar pattern whereby conference papers are presented in order under their authors' names has not been adopted here. Instead the manuscripts have been combined in a manner that allows the important themes to be retained, yet developed into a cohesive whole. Repetition is avoided by combining relevant matter from different contributors into newly formed chapters. However, the content generated by the original speaker is preceded by his or her name in parentheses, thus *(Smith)*; some small, unmarked sections of text are of editorial origin. In this way, it has been possible to produce a condensed account which allows the reader to assimilate readily the important issues that a geographically widespread group of experts and delegates raised and discussed. The account also provides a synopsis of the scientific background which will be the basis for making the moves that are needed to effect the desired changes.

The term 'evolution' has been chosen to encapsulate these considerations within the title of the book. Evolution implies a gradual change from one thing to another, in this case from dental treatment to oral health. While some might argue that 'oral health' should have featured in the title rather than 'dental care', the fact is that most of the current oral health personnel are dentists or their auxiliary staff, and it is to these people and other medical workers that this book is primarily directed, together with academics, health services personnel and administrators, as well as research workers in dental and allied fields.

Ultimately it is the non-specialist, the consumer, the person-in-the-street, who stands to gain most by the evolutionary trends described here. It is therefore hoped that this book may prove accessible to those many individuals whose interaction and constructive criticism will be essential if the evolutionary process is to be fulfilled during the lifetimes of some present members of our global society.

RJE
Bristol
August 1989

Acknowledgements

Grateful thanks go to Mentadent Preventive Dental Care for generous sponsorship of the Bristol '88 World Dental Conference, making it possible for speakers to be invited from so many distant parts of the world. Editorial assistance in the task of reducing the record of the conference to manageable proportions was provided by Dr M.B. Edwards. The Appendix is reproduced by kind permission of the editor of the *British Dental Journal*. The contents of M.C. Downer's contribution represent the author's views alone and in no way commit the Department of Health. Work reported by N.B. Pitts was supported by the Chief Scientist Office of the Scottish Home and Health Department. The following contributors acknowledge the generous assistance of colleagues (and sponsors) as follows: S. Warnakulasuriya and A.Ekanayake – Lever Brothers (Cey) Ltd., Mrs Chandani Nanayakkara and Mr Asange Karunaratne; N.W. Johnson – colleagues in the MRC Dental Research Unit, Periodontal Disease Programme; K.L. Lester – Drs R. Bryant, R.J.F. Butler, R. Widmer, and Professor A.J. Spencer.

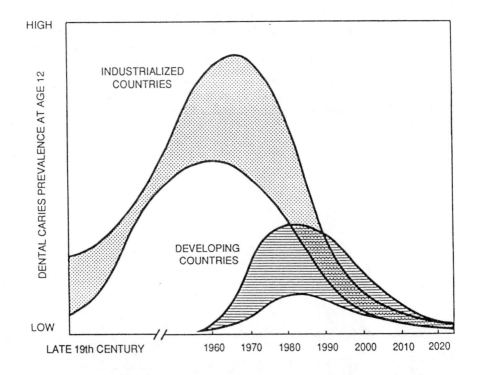

Schematic representation of the global prevalence of dental caries at age 12 years since the late nineteenth century, with a forecast into the first quarter of the twenty-first century. The upper and lower limits of the shaded areas (which have not been corrected for population size) give an idea of the ranges of prevalence found across different regions of the world; these fall broadly into two groups – industrialized countries and developing countries. While caries prevalence at age 12 is still rising in some developing countries, in others the fall has already set in, thereby giving considerable grounds for optimism that the disease can be controlled to trivial levels on a global scale within the foreseeable future.

1
Introduction

Our world is made artificially small by diverse means of communication. By these means the most developed countries often appear to export images of affluence, success and satisfaction, not least in matters of health. In much the same way they seem almost to require the less developed to generate reciprocal images of poverty, disease and despair. Neither set of images is accurate, but undoubtedly the highly industrialized nations do have economic muscle – they can influence or even coerce the less strong into accepting alien 'solutions' to what they (the strong) choose to define as 'problems'. But to do so is often to ignore what is appropriate to the needs of a developing country and what pertains to the essence of its culture. Nowhere is the need for appropriateness more clear than in health services.

Globally, oral health has not escaped evaluation for appropriateness. As explained in the Preface, to acknowledge and explore this process was one reason for holding the conference upon which this book is based. In fact, the meeting was not long under way before a speaker from the Indian subcontinent applied a general and frequently articulated question to the specifics of oral health care: 'What can we learn from the follies of the West?' At least part of an answer may be found within these pages.

In the space of two paragraphs a crop of problematical definitions has already been sown. On what scale and by what right may a country be regarded as 'developed', and which of these are 'industrialized' or ultimately 'post-industrialized'? There are incomplete, quantitative answers to these questions but these do not remove all the difficulties, and precision in usage of these terms is not claimed here. Many of the conference speakers used 'Western', or 'in the West' in the context of economic progress and success. They were not ignorant of achievements in the Far East or unaware of the coming of what many term the 'Pacific century'. Rather they followed a convention that may now be inaccurate and, to some, redolent of inappropriate value judgements, but which remains illustrative. Others preferred the terms 'developing' and 'developed', perhaps because these sound more neutral.

In communicating what for the most part is the conceptual basis of the conference, the editor has been happy to stick to generalities, not least in the hope of reaching as broad a readership as possible. Only one Figure (facing this page) was deemed essential, and references have been pared away to a minimum. The single Figure illustrates a basic premise that is later expanded. This is that the prevalence of dental caries is generally declining in developed countries and is increasing (sometimes with alarming rapidity) or has the

1

potential to increase in the developing world. In a sense, the core of this book forms around the significance of this observation both to regions directly afflicted by the problem and to the developed countries, which have responded to their version of this 'epidemic' in the past. But this is not to say that the periodontal diseases, anomalies of occlusion, and oral mucosal diseases have not been considered in detail and, where necessary, in a critical fashion. Rather, it seems – and here we begin with a conclusion – that caries (and oral cancer) may continue to have the greater impact on strategies for oral health care, especially in developing counties.

There are times when anecdote may lend a cutting edge to the traditional but too often turgid objectivity of scientific communications. The reasons for selecting Maria's story as a starting point should be self-evident.

MARIA'S STORY

(Hobdell) Maria was born in 1975 in a small village just outside the tiny market town of Montepuez in Cabo Delgado Province, Mozambique. She was the eldest of 10 children. Her family lived on their own plot of land near to a small stream that provided them with water. Her father had gone to work in the kapok plantations in the next province and came home only once a year; Maria's brothers and sisters all had birthdays about nine months after his annual holiday.

Maria was a happy child, and as her father's salary was raised, she eventually had money to buy Fanta and toffees. But one day, when she was about 10 years old, she woke up with a pain in her tooth. She had never had this before, but went off to school thinking it was a growing pain and would go away. It stayed and got worse. Her mother looked in her mouth to find a big black hole in one of her bottom teeth. They went and spoke with the neighbours who suggested they dig up and grind a local root and put the powder in the hole. They did this and Maria got some relief. The incident was forgotten until the same thing happened on the other side of her mouth. They repeated the process, as it had worked before, but this time the relief was only short-lived.

Maria woke one morning with a swollen, flushed and painful face; more neighbourly consultation followed. It was the general opinion that Maria had got worms in her teeth. The only person who could help was the traditional healer in the next village. No school for Maria that day: she and her mother trudged stoically off to find the healer outside his hut. They talked about the weather and the crops and then about Maria's face and teeth. He suggested smoking the worms out, so he went inside his hut and came back with a dried-milk tin full of twigs. With these he built a fire and sat Maria opposite himself with the fire between them. He then took a long bamboo pole and started to blow the smoke gently across at Maria's face. Her eyes streaming, Maria gradually began to feel the pain getting less. After a while the fire died

2

down, so Maria's mother paid the healer and they went back home. Maria's face never returned to normal but there was little pain so she went back to school for a few weeks.

Then it all started again. This time neighbourly consultation revealed that a new 'tooth doctor' had arrived at the little hospital in Montepuez. So Maria and her mother went to seek his advice. They got there as João was cleaning up after his morning's work. He looked at Maria's fat face and said she should have a series of antibiotic injections. Poor little Maria had never had an injection in her life. The smallpox eradication team had simply 'shot' with a dermojet in the arm, so when he asked her to bare her bottom she was shocked. However, her mother said she must. João, meanwhile, was explaining that he would be as gentle as possible but as he only had three re-usable needles, which were quite old, it might hurt a little. Maria was brave but it took a lot not to cry out as the needle went in. João said they must return each day for the next four days.

The next day's injection was worse, either because Maria was more tense, knowing what was to happen, or it could have been an even blunter needle. The third day was the worst and poor Maria let out a terrible yell as the needle went in. But on the fourth day when she woke she felt better and it was relatively easy for her to persuade her mother not to go back, for she was all behind in fetching water, washing the clothes and tending the family fields. Maria felt she was cured. But her hopes were dashed when, some weeks later, she woke to find her mouth worse than ever. Both sides of her neck were swollen and she could hardly lift her head. Her mother took one look and said they must go back to João.

João remembered Maria and quite understood why they had not returned before. Unfortunately, he explained, he was completely out of any antibiotics as the lorry from Maputo had gone off the road and all the drugs were lost. He advised them that Maria was indeed very ill and must get treatment. He suggested that they take the bus to Pemba, the provincial capital, and go to the hospital there. They just managed to cram themselves into the lopsided vehicle as it stood at the bus depot. It had no windscreen and moved slowly along the road in a crabwise fashion, and they got to Pemba long after the outpatient department had shut. So they slept the night on a bench waiting in line with others who had also made the tiring journey.

In the morning Maria was delirious and the doctor immediately said she must be admitted. Poor Maria, who had never been away from home and had never slept in a bed with sheets or in a room with a ceiling, felt terrible. Her mother was torn between staying with her or going back to look after her other children. In the end she had to leave Maria behind, not knowing it would be over a year before she saw her again. The doctors tried and tried to control Maria's infection, but each time they seemed to be on top of it the bacteria developed resistance to their drugs, which were never in a properly continuous supply. In the end they decided that Maria had to go to the capital, Maputo. Then more problems: no transport was available; the roads were impassable and anyway it would take too long for such a sick child. She had to be sent by plane.

So Maria arrived in the Central Hospital in Maputo. She was a small frightened 10-year-old sitting in the old-fashioned upright dental chair, her little head barely reaching the head rest. She was dressed in a tattered pale-blue hospital nightdress, the top of which was soaked in pus that dribbled from two scarlet sinuses, one on each side of her neck. The swellings in her neck were complemented by the absence of all her lower teeth and, in their place, there were fragments of white sequestrated bone poking through the oral mucosa and surrounded by pus.

She had osteomyelitis of the mandible extending from coronoid process to coronoid process. She was given extensive antibiotic therapy over a prolonged period, supported by local curettage and cleaning. Eventually no more sequestra separated and the mucosa healed, leaving her with a toothless jaw of a shape and size that might be found in someone long edentulous and of advanced years. A complete lower denture was constructed and she was sent home to her village in the far north of the country, a journey equivalent to travelling from Edinburgh to Gibraltar.

This illustration has been taken from one of the poorest nations of the world. In countries like Mozambique oral health care must, of necessity, take a relatively minute share of human and physical resources. Indeed, for the majority of the world, any type of professional oral health care remains simply a remote possibility. But it is not just the question of how human and economic resources may be redistributed to take account of such inequalities that makes Maria's story immediately relevant to all health care providers, whether from rich or poor countries. The picture of her plight is a miniature of how and why dental disease evolved in the past in those parts of the world where now, by and large, it is taken for granted. Such 'living history' gives an unavoidable opportunity for objective assessment, with hindsight, of the successes and failures of modern dentistry. Without a long, hard look at the causes and implications of Maria's plight, neither effective solutions to it nor sensible plans for the future of oral health care in the developed world are likely to emerge.

The bare bones of such an analysis emerge in Chapter 2. At this stage it should suffice to say that the challenge for modern dentistry, wherever it is practised, is to devise scientifically sound, socially acceptable and economically viable ways of preventing and treating common oral diseases. The uniform content and provision of oral health care in industrialized countries, focused as it is on surgery, certainly does not preclude the possibility that there might be more appropriate alternatives for those countries not geared to sustaining such specialized and demanding activities. Indeed it can be argued that it is anachronistic even for industrialized countries to continue to use nineteenth century technology – drilling and filling; scaling and polishing – to combat caries and periodontal diseases.

2
Dental care, past and present – success or failure?

(Pinto) A host of variables fosters the appearance of oral diseases in any community. Of major importance are the extent of economic development, the type of government organization, the educational level of the population and the cultural standards and traditions that condition personal or collective patterns of diet and hygiene. In relation to such factors, a community tends to become burdened by specific sets of oral diseases, each with its own level of severity and incidence, strongly conditioned by environmental and social determinants.

Although there may thus be diverse patterns of disease, it would seem obvious that oral health care needs and the provision of services are but two faces of the same coin, yet in reality each often tends to follow a different path. The situation today is that relatively larger numbers of dentists are found in countries where the population has reached (either currently or in the recent past) high levels of dental caries – even though the incidence of disease is now falling. It is a paradox that economically strong and prosperous dental practice has come to coexist with a high prevalence of this disease.

This book began with an illustrative story from Mozambique. To take another example from the developing world, the layman may ask why, in Ethiopia, a country with the world's lowest annual *per capita* income (US$ 110), most children are free from dental caries, while in West Germany (US$ 10 940 *per capita*) this disease still affects so many. The answer is straightforward: caries is not an 'ailment of poverty', as are many transmissible diseases and those that come from malnutrition; rather it is an outcome of economic development and a sequel to rising sugar consumption. Economic development has also brought more dentists, but they have not been able to prevent the initiation and spread of caries for, as will be discussed in detail later, they have been dedicated almost exclusively to treatment-based services, often tailored only to those who can afford them.

Especially with regard to the prevalence of caries in children and young people, today's world can be roughly divided into three large groups:

– the poorer nations of the developing world in which traditionally low levels of caries have started to rise in line with industrialization;

– those developing countries that have made definite economic progress but which are, in general, undergoing a period of severe economic crisis and which are at the top of the world caries statistics (and apparently unable to change their own epidemiological picture);

5

— the richest nations, which have reached high levels of caries in the past but which have gradually managed to control the problem.

It is realistic to examine the global prevalence of caries at 12 years of age in relation to the availability of dentists, income levels and sugar consumption, in order to obtain a more detailed picture. In 1985, low-income nations, comprising nearly two-thirds of the world population, had about 8 per cent of the available dentists and low levels of both sugar consumption and caries (although there are now strong indications that the disease is on the increase). In the low-income countries of Asia, there were, on average, some 47 760 individuals to one dentist. However, the index of decayed, missing and filled teeth for these people was as yet among the lowest in the world – a mean of 2.18 teeth in 12-year-old children – second only to Africa. The picture was varied in the middle-income nations but, the other extreme, high-income nations, comprising 26 per cent of the world population and with 68 per cent of the dentists, have only recently had decreasing levels of caries, and of significant proportions only since the middle of the last decade. These industrialized countries have at least a three-fold greater mean daily sugar supply *per capita* than the low-income areas of Africa and Asia. However, the sugar supply of the developed countries is similar now to that of developing, middle-income countries, such as in Central and South America, where dentists are not numerous and caries is highly prevalent.

Globally there was a rise of about 10 per cent in sugar consumption between 1975 and 1985, the most significant increases being in Asia (60 per cent) and Africa (20 per cent). Estimates for 1985–8 suggest a slight fall in consumption around the world, despite the opposing trend in Asia and Africa. Some significant decreases in sugar intake have also occurred, led by a 22 per cent reduction in North America. World sugar production has, however, been steadily increasing, albeit at a rate below population growth during the last three years.

The established response to rising levels of caries has been to increase the number of dentists and strengthen dental practice. The need for any response at all probably reflects the fact that caries may have acute effects, generally involving pain. This is in contrast to the periodontal diseases, which are normally chronic and pain-free. Indeed, periodontal diseases, which have affected humankind since early times, appeared to gain attention and status in the dental health league only when caries began to be curbed in industrialized countries.

(*Tala*) It was in the early years of the nineteenth century that the incidence of caries started to rise rapidly in the Western world, as can be inferred from the Figure (facing p. 1). The reasons for that rise were unknown at the time. This 'epidemic' coincided with the invention of silver–tin amalgam for use as a filling material, thus making restoration an acceptable alternative to the traditional extraction. The 'filling philosophy' soon spread widely and a large number of dental faculties were established. The alarming amount of caries among children resulted in the formation of school dental programmes in the late 1800s and early 1900s, but the incidence of the disease rose much faster than the capacity of dentists to treat it. Governments became aware of the problem and goals for the education of dentists were set.

Today it may reasonably be argued that most of these early programmes failed. Indeed it is pertinent to ask what has the 'nineteenth century technology', referred to at the end of Chapter 1, achieved overall in combating dental caries and periodontal diseases? Despite huge financial investment in the industrialized countries, the traditional approach of reparative and restorative dentistry has clearly not resulted in excellent oral health. In the Nordic countries and the UK a large proportion of adults, at least until very recently, still ultimately lost all their natural teeth. In Finland, even in the early 1980s, the most common status for permanent teeth among the entire population was 'missing' and this at a time when the country was just about to reach the goal of one dentist for every 1000 persons in the population. A high prevalence of filled teeth was another typical feature.

Because of the irreversible nature of restorative treatment, the limits for improvement in the dental health of a population, when assessed in terms of missing or filled teeth, are set for many decades to come. At least 50 years are needed before it would be even theoretically possible to have most members of a seriously affected population with totally sound (unfilled) teeth.

On the other hand, dental science has advanced a number of effective preventive methods, based upon breakthroughs that include:

- water fluoridation, from 1945;

- Stephan's pH curve, 1945;

- Vipeholm sugar studies, 1952;

- fissure sealants, from 1952;

- germfree animal studies, from 1959;

- chlorhexidine, from 1970;

- sugar substitute studies, from 1974.

The important point is that preventive methods, and their scientific base, have been established for many years but without their widespread implementation. Unfortunately, it is mostly ethical and legal controversy that has prevented large numbers of people from receiving the substantial benefits offered by fluoridation of public water supplies.

How then did the evident improvements in oral health in most developed countries actually come about? *(Sheiham)* Many would argue that they are due mainly to preventive action taken by individuals and government rather than to increased availability of dental manpower. Falling levels of caries have certainly occurred in countries both with and without preventive schemes organized at the professional level. For example, such changes are found in England, which has had few schemes for fluoride rinsing or professionally applied topical fluoride and little systematic dental health education, as well as relatively few general dental practitioners using specific preventive measures such as fissure sealants. And the caries rate is lower in England than in Scandinavian countries, which do have large-scale fluoride rinsing and dental health education programmes.

To some extent the successes and failures of oral health care in the developing world reflect the same attitudes and problems as in the developed countries because of the acquisition of 'Western' methods (*see* p. 11 and 62). *(Lembariti)* In developing countries, however, a further critical determinant of oral health policy and strategy development is the availability of personnel (including those potentially available for training). This may be severely limited by factors such as widespread illiteracy and a dearth of physical resources. These factors assume special significance in areas where there is no tradition of centrally organized and integrated health services.

(Sardo Infirri) The present arrangements for oral care services result in the majority of dentists throughout the world being located in urban areas. In the towns and cities of developing countries there are usually limited services available in the public sector, but private practice flourishes autonomously for those who can afford it. Care in the public services is often severely restricted by poor or malfunctioning equipment, and a lack of instruments, materials and drugs; the staff are often badly paid in comparison with the financial rewards of private practice. This combination of factors frequently results in low morale and motivation. Teeth with minor lesions are often extracted because that is the only treatment available. Some kind of prosthesis may then be offered by the same care provider, but as part of a second job as a private practitioner.

In rural areas of most developing countries, dentists are almost unknown – and it is clear that the majority of carious or infected teeth are not even extracted. Rather the diseases progress, causing intermittent pain that the owner of the tooth manages by avoiding the use of the affected area of the mouth. Only if extreme pain or severe infection develop is an attempt made to find dental treatment, as exemplified by Maria's story in Chapter 1. This is frequently provided by a general health worker or a traditional healer in private practice. At this stage, the treatment is usually costly when counted in terms of loss of income and productivity, travel expenses and dental fees, which may be as high as those charged by a dentist in an urban area. It is also more likely that debilitating or even life-threatening conditions will be allowed to develop through postponement of effective care at this stage.

In an effort to ensure that services are more equitably spread, some countries have introduced compulsory service in rural areas for all dentists.

However, where such policies have not been backed up by effective resources and referral possibilities, they have not worked well. This may partly explain the large differences in dental status in middle age shown by national oral health surveys in two parts of South East Asia: both have a similar and low level of caries among 12-year-olds but, by the age of 35–44 years, adults on average have about 5 missing teeth where there is compulsory rural service, compared with about 2.5 where such a service does not exist. While there may, of course, be geographical and lifestyle factors involved, much of the difference is probably the result of the extraction of teeth with relatively minor lesions where the service exists to carry this out. Certainly, the compulsory deployment of dentists does not seem to have delivered the conservative care that might have been expected and that could largely have eliminated loss of teeth.

(Pinto) In general terms, dentistry has evolved gradually in the developing world from two basic components: an inescapable duty to provide basic dental care to meet the real demands of individuals in the lower income brackets; and a corporate pressure for job places exercised by dentists, a well-structured group within the society. The outcome is that oral diseases, after reaching high or very high levels (as in many parts of South America), are maintained without significant change at a point of potentially unstable equilibrium. Here the population, plagued by so many different but vital difficulties, seems to accept that such diseases and their sequelae of extractions and protheses are either unavoidable facts of life or natural consequences of financial hardship. And, at the end of the disease process, as described above, the attention of specialists may be required, bringing with them costs that are unsustainable, both for the individuals and for the service.

It has already been noted that oral health care services tend to have little impact when they have been developed within traditional models, that is when they are treatment-based and function to meet a demand conditioned by extant problems. Indeed, whenever a country, region or locality selects the treatment-based system, and whenever a service or programme limits its scope to the provision of job places, improvement of community health services is virtually unattainable. The availability of reasonably well-distributed services in sufficient quantity is just not enough. In order actually to benefit a population's health, the services need to be properly organized and sufficiently funded. Funding through taxes appears to be the most suitable method for programmes to cover large populations.

Truly private dental practice, based on market conditions, is usually favoured by dental professionals, but its application is, or course, restricted to individuals who can afford the services. In countries lacking economic development, these individuals are generally a minority comprising 10–30 per cent of the population; making such services universally available is unthinkable. The other well-tried model (as in the UK) is that of indirect provision of services, generally financed by social security arrangements and offered by dentists in their own practices. This may entail high costs due to the presence of a third party between the patient and the professional. In addition, it frequently emphasizes a treatment-based approach and is some-times subject to fraud. Though some industrialized countries have obtained 'satisfactory' results from these two models, neither has been shown able to improve the epidemiological picture in the developing world. The alternative arrangement, whereby the dentist is hired and paid a salary, does not dis-criminate so much against potential users who lack the means to pay, and constitutes, in principle, the avenue for provision of appropriate services to all.

AN OVERVIEW OF ORAL HEALTH TODAY

(Barmes) The first conclusion that may be drawn is very simple: extraction of the tooth as the easiest solution for any dental problem has declined vastly in developed countries – the increasing tendency for older people to retain teeth bears witness to this encouraging trend. Few will doubt that this important change stems mostly from social pressure, and it serves to emphas-ize the importance of the interaction between providers and consumers. Directly related to the declining use of extractions is the prosthetic option. The available information suggests that, despite an increase in the provision of fixed prostheses, the emphasis placed on such procedures is far less in practice than would be ideal. Even where such emphasis is strong, the precision and quality of the treatment may leave much to be desired. There is at present considerable reluctance (and with good reason) to go further into the techniques of prosthetic implants and tissue integration.

The first phase of the International Collaborative Study of Oral Health Systems in industrialized countries showed that most methods examined in the 1970s had failed, by a considerable margin, to convert the 'decayed' component of the decayed, missing and filled index to 'filled' at any of the ages studied (8–9, 13–14 and 35–44 years). However, there were notable exceptions, such as for the 13–14 year age groups in New Zealand, with its well-organized and enthusiastic school dental service. Caries prevalence was already declining in many of the countries studied and it would be comforting to think that the unrestored 'decayed' factor signified planned non-interven-tion, based upon careful application of predetermined criteria. But there was no indication that this was the case – the unrestored component simply signified lack of coverage through consumer or provider omission.

The use of fissure sealants and the non-intervention approach to early caries, together with other less tissue-destructive restorative techniques (*see* Chapter 3), are now being taught, but it is clear that the 'cutting and filling' response to a diagnosis of caries remains strong, especially among prac-titioners who graduated before the last 5 to 10 years. It may, therefore, be suspected that there has been considerable over-intervention for those who visit dental practices, though most of this was not at variance with what the practitioners were taught. There remains, of course, the opposite problem – that of non-users of dental services, for whom lesions which need intervention are not receiving appropriate treatment.

Similar to the 'cutting and filling' response, the tendency to scale routinely where calculus is detected probably predominates over efforts to instil adequate oral hygiene first and to follow up with selective scaling later. It is difficult to tell how far the popularity of non-surgical versus surgical intervention has developed in the management of destructive periodontal conditions, but it is likely that there still is a tendency to over-use the surgical approach in industrialized countries.

Orthodontics is the rich and at the same time the poor relation of the above: rich because the practice of orthodontics has increased, at high cost, for a growing clientele in industrialized countries; poor because no one has truly come to grips with how it should be handled. Orthodontics has polarized thinking about oral health care more than any other specialty. Those in favour recommend more and more of it at increasing levels of sophistication, for an ever-increasing range of ages. Those who are against see it almost as a fashion trade for both the rich consumers and the affluent and elite practitioners, with relevance for those in true need whatever their circumstances, but a purely cosmetic luxury for the others. Clearly, reality fits neither of these extremes. For the present, there appears to be a cocktail of over- and under-intervention in orthodontics, the pressing problem being to find out what is objectively relevant to treatment needs (*see* Chapter 3.).

Care of other oral conditions seems often to remain firmly ensconced in '*ad hoc*-ery'. From society to society, oral health personnel involve themselves, to a greater or lesser extent, in surgery for benign and malignant growths and in the management of the less common diseases and conditions of the mouth, which are often related to systemic factors. There is every indication that these conditions are growing in importance, in line with greater emphasis on the control of cross-infection in dental practice, and linked with more refined notions of medical fitness for dental treatment (*see* Chapter 3).

In developing countries the current responses to oral diseases are generally similar to those in the industrialized countries, because the personnel involved has either been trained in industrialized countries (*see* p. 62), or in local schools with curricula largely adopted from industrialized countries and usually from one, two, or more decades in the past. The differences in oral health care in these countries are therefore related to oral health status and trends, availability of personnel and logistics. The fact that a number of developing countries still have caries levels no greater than a mean of 1 decayed, missing or filled tooth per 12-year-old child means that the 'cutting and filling' response is even less relevant, although it is definitely alive and well in such countries. However, communities with a mean of between 2 to 4 decayed, missing or filled teeth at 12 years of age regularly record mean values for 'filled' teeth of 0.1–0.2, a clear indication of lack of personnel and facilities. The high prevalence of gingival bleeding and calculus, and yet usually low prevalence of destructive forms of periodontal disease, might have prompted the 'hygiene first' response, but it appears that, ironically, the prophylaxis (scaling) response to the detection of calculus is even more Pavlovian than in the industrialized countries.

(Sardo Infirri) It is salutary to consider the estimated treatment needs over a lifetime for the populations of developing countries. This can be quantified in terms of the extractions likely to be needed because of severe caries or periodontal diseases. Statistics in the World Health Organization Global Oral Data Bank, combined with the United Nations population estimates for 1985, suggest that about 36 per cent of these populations (some 1250 million people) will require three or fewer extractions in a lifetime, and 64 per cent (2400 million people) will need four or more extractions. This calculation indicates that, perhaps, 300 million extractions will be needed each year. If we assume that a dentist working only as an 'extractor' could remove about 5000 teeth per year, then 60 000 dentists would be needed. As there are more than 185 000 dentists working in developing countries there would appear to be adequate manpower to give this essential pain relief and emergency care, provided that they do nothing else but extract (which they do not) and that they are equally distributed throughout the global population, which, of course, again they are not.

3
Current understanding of oral diseases and abnormalities

So far, general aspects of oral health care provision have been examined; details of new approaches are described in Chapter 4. In the present chapter, oral diseases and other abnormalities, such as malocclusion, are considered in greater detail – the context being recent advances in understanding and implications for their management.

PERIODONTAL DISEASES

(Pilot) Destructive periodontal diseases are currently thought to progress in periodic, relatively short episodes of rapid tissue destruction, sometimes followed by a degree of repair, and mostly by prolonged periods of quiescence. Loss of periodontal attachment is not evenly distributed within the dentition, nor in populations. Some people have frequent episodes of active disease at many sites in their mouths – they constitute a rapidly progressing (high-risk) group. Others experience far less active disease, with signs of gingivitis and maybe some pocketing, but with not much attachment loss over prolonged periods. These low-risk people have slowly developing periodontal diseases.

(Cutress) Recently the World Health Organization and the Fédération Dentaire Internationale developed a procedure, the Community Periodontal Index of Treatment Needs (CPITN), for assessing periodontal conditions and identifying the needs of populations and individuals for periodontal care.[1] This index removes some of the mystique surrounding periodontal diseases and their treatment, and offers a realistic procedure for preliminary diagnostic screening of individuals and population groups and for rationalizing treatment needs, both at the community level and in dental practice. It is simple, quick to apply and has international uniformity.

The CPITN is compatible with current concepts of disease progression and control. It confines clinical observations to the criteria most relevant to treatment needs: pockets, gingival inflammation (identified by bleeding on gentle probing), calculus and other plaque-retentive factors. Assessment of past and present deviations from health, such as gingival recession, tooth mobility and loss of attachment, are considered less relevant to improving periodontal health.[2]

A function of CPITN screening is to stream individuals to their appropriate level of care: self-care, dental auxiliary, practitioner or specialist (*see* p.

84). Indeed, its primary value is in co-ordinating a realistic approach to a condition that has largely been ignored in the past. It is, of course, acknowledged that social, economic, personnel and other factors will influence decisions on priorities concerning management of the diseases so identified.[3]

Full details of the CPITN examination are readily available: the highest score in each sextant of the dentition is determined, and in epidemiological surveys of adults, only 10 index teeth are scored, which underestimates the total need by about 20 per cent. For general practice, all teeth should be examined, but only the highest score is recorded for each sextant. A special ball-ended CPITN probe has been designed for easy identification of calculus, pocket depths and bleeding. The average time for a CPITN assessment is three to four minutes.

The highest of the following codes for each index tooth is scored as follows:

Code 0	Healthy periodontal tissues.
Code 1	Gingival bleeding following gentle probing.
Code 2	Supra- or subgingival calculus or defective margin of restoration causing plaque retention.
Code 3	Pathological pocket 4–5 mm deep.
Code 4	Pathological pocket 6 mm or deeper.

Codes 1–4 indicate these three general levels of treatment needs:

Treatment need 1	Need for improved oral hygiene (Code 1 scored).
Treatment need 2	Need for improved oral hygiene and removal of calculus and/or defective margins of restorations (Codes 2 or 3 scored).
Treatment need 3	Need for improved oral hygiene and complex periodontal care (Code 4 scored).

This last level is considered as tertiary prevention (*see* p. 84), which is necessary to prevent progression of advanced disease and tooth loss. It requires special clinical skills and may involve pocket eradication in addition to scaling and oral hygiene instruction.

CPITN is increasingly being adopted as a successful method for promoting awareness of periodontal diseases on a mass scale. Organized promotion of periodontal health is under way in various countries including the UK, USA, Finland, Sri Lanka, New Zealand, Italy, Portugal and Colombia. In the UK and New Zealand, periodontal awareness programmes include a Gum Health Plan (*see* also p. 59), which comprises self-assessment, a self-help guide, and free educational and promotional material on request. In the UK a pilot study has revealed a favourable response from more than 80 per cent of interested general dental practitioners.

The epidemiological picture

(*Pilot*) Via the World Health Organization Global Oral Data Bank, the results of CPITN surveys from many countries around the world now permit a realistic picture of periodontal diseases and their implications at the community level.

For adolescents, bleeding on probing has been found very commonly in some surveys, but the most frequent item in this age group has been calculus with or without bleeding (CPITN score 2). Shallow pocketing (of 4 or 5 mm) has generally affected only a minority of the sample, and then only in one or two sextants. Adults aged 35–44 years with completely healthy periodontal tissues are virtually non-existent, calculus and shallow pocketing being the most frequent conditions. Except in a few studies, the percentages of persons with deep pockets (6 mm and deeper) and the mean number of sextants per person with them have been small (*see* 'high-risk groups' below). Tooth loss because of periodontal diseases has not often been encountered in adults around 40 years of age.

(*Johnson*) The CPITN may have limitations, notably the absence of information on attachment level and a restriction to the use of sample index teeth in some surveys, but the growing mass of CPITN data world-wide clearly supports the view that only a relatively small minority of the population is at risk of developing destructive disease.[4] Those from Italy and from the Philippines provide good examples: the 'worst' CPITN score (4) was found in less than 20 per cent of 35–64-year-olds in Italy and in a mere 4 per cent of 45–85-year-olds in the Philippines. In both surveys, on average, less than 1 per cent of the population was edentulous, and the high scores affected substantially less than one sextant. If the distribution of the disease were to be examined in detail in these populations, most people with high scores would probably be found to have only one site with this degree of pocketing and a minority of individuals would account for most of the deep pockets recorded.

(*Pilot*) The conclusion must therefore be that, for the large majority of people in most of the populations observed, the progress of destructive periodontal diseases has been slow and seems to be compatible with the retention of a natural dentition until at least the age of 50 years. And this despite the high prevalence of gingivitis and periodontitis. This conclusion provides a much more optimistic outlook than hitherto, even though periodontal conditions for which specific intervention (such as oral hygiene instruction and scaling) might be considered are widespread around the world. While there are few global data concerning people over about 50 years of age, it should be appreciated that life expectancy is relatively low in developing countries, and that oral health can be expected to improve along with improvements in general health, hygiene and living conditions (as has happened in developed countries).

It is important to note that the previously assumed differences between industrialized and developing countries for the prevalence and severity of periodontal diseases have not been reflected in the global statistics. There have, however, been marked differences between such countries in the estimated levels of edentulousness, few people being found without teeth in the developing countries. The relatively high levels of edentulousness that have been reported in industrialized countries appear, as has been noted in Chapter 2, to reflect a lack of success with the management of caries and restorative treatment.

The question arises, has there been a real improvement in the periodontal condition globally or is the problem now better investigated and understood? It seems that the latter is largely the case, although there is no doubt that oral hygiene has been improved over the last few decades in a number of countries. The numbers of children with overt gingivitis have decreased in some industrialized countries, and the periodontal condition of adults has improved. Sales of toothpaste and toothbrushes have increased; there is even concern about an increase in toothbrush trauma to the teeth in children and adolescents.

With hindsight, it is easy to give a number of explanations for misunderstandings about the true incidence of periodontal diseases. Early investigations of reasons for tooth loss contain methodological flaws in the selection of experimental groups and in diagnostic criteria. There has also been some 'brainwashing' by averages: reports on *mean* periodontal attachment loss *per year* do not show the sites where the periodontal tissues are breaking down at a much faster rate than average, nor the distribution and numbers of the affected persons (including those who are, in fact, in the high-risk category). Persons and sites with no attachment loss at all are also obscured by mean figures. Furthermore, in the early epidemiological surveys, any deviation from the ideal was recorded and implicitly considered as disease. Such records have definite value in experimental clinical trials, but in population studies they can easily lead to an over-estimation of treatment needs. Lastly, it should be appreciated that it is unrealistic to define as health the complete absence of symptoms or of any deviation from the ideal. Health is a relative entity and, according to a World Health Organization definition, it should be such as to enable a socially and economically productive life. For an older person, a functioning natural dentition is *not* a set of 32 teeth, caries-free, in perfect alignment and with nice gingiva up to the cementum–enamel junction, but something better expressed as 'enough teeth to smile and enough molars to chew'; or, more technically, a stable, functional contact between the upper and the lower jaws. Such is now a realistic and generally attainable goal at the community level. However, there are still professional and community barriers to the provision and acceptance of periodontal care, including a public lack of perception of the symptoms and a low priority for treatment by many dental practitioners.

Problems of classification

(Johnson) There are many different types of inflammatory periodontal disease for which there may be different aetiologies, and certainly there are very different host predisposing and resistance factors. No entirely satisfactory classification exists because all these factors are insufficiently understood. Current practice tends to use clinical descriptors (e.g. gingivitis or periodontitis), age of onset, rate of progression, and site distribution within the mouth as the basis for subdivision. Reference is commonly made to 'entities' such as childhood gingivitis, localized juvenile periodontitis, rapidly progressive adult periodontitis and chronic adult periodontitis, but most of these are poorly defined.

Though gingivitis is universal, or nearly so, in many populations, most forms of the disease are self-limiting and reversible. Tooth support and function are not compromised by gingivitis and so its importance in public health terms remains low. The contemporary view is that one must separate the presence of overt gingivitis from any preconceived notion that disease will inevitably affect the deeper tissues. In other words, gingivitis and destructive periodontitis appear not to have the strong causal inter-relationship it was once thought they had. Such longitudinal data as are available provide no evidence for progression of gingivitis to destructive periodontitis, and severe periodontal breakdown often occurs in the absence of marked gingivitis – for example, in juvenile periodontitis and so-called rapidly progressive adult periodontitis. Indeed gingivitis may best be regarded as the normal day-to-day functioning of the host response, not as a harbinger of inevitable periodontal destruction. If a population can be moved towards greater awareness of periodontal health and disease and towards more effective oral hygiene, it should be possible to shift most people away from overt gingivitis, whatever its ultimate relationship with 'destructive periodontitis'.

High-risk groups

The proportion of a population at high risk of periodontal breakdown of sufficient extent and severity to cause concern because of pain, functional or aesthetic deterioration inevitably depends upon the definitions employed. Gingival crevice depths of six or more millimetres and loss of periodontal attachment of four or more millimetres may be considered as substantial levels of periodontal breakdown; using these to define an 'at-risk' threshold, a prevalence figure of 7–15 per cent has emerged with remarkable consistency in many recent surveys in industrialized and developing countries.

However, current understanding of the natural history of destructive periodontitis is poor. Longitudinal studies (studies conducted over a period of time) are required but these are costly and it takes decades before useful results are produced. The work of Loe and his colleagues[5] concerning Sri Lankan tea-estate labourers is thus of seminal importance. This clearly demonstrated, over 15 years, rapidly, moderately and non-progressive disease in groups representing 8, 81 and 11 per cent of the population respectively. A spectrum of disease progression was found, and this was not related to levels of oral hygiene, calculus or gingivitis. There is an implication here of the importance of host factors; this is a population with chronic under-nutrition and a high level of intercurrent disease.

The ability to identify high-risk individuals in advance would be a major breakthrough, as would be methods for detecting individual periodontal sites that were susceptible to breakdown, or were undergoing a phase of active disease. There is much current research in this area; encouraging progress is being made but, before putative markers can be brought into routine clinical practice, each needs to be evaluated in careful (and inevitably lengthy) longitudinal studies designed to assess reproducibility, reliability, sensitivity and specificity. A distinction should also be made between *predictors* of future breakdown and *indicators* of current disease activity, though similar disease *markers* may be sought for both purposes. Some of the current understanding of these areas is now summarized; (readers not seeking precise details at this stage may choose to advance to p. 23).

Predisposing factors

Genetic and racial predisposition. The familial occurrence of juvenile periodontitis is well known and this appears to be inherited as an autosomal recessive with full penetrance. Screening of relatives should, therefore, always be undertaken when a case is diagnosed. The genetic linkage is consistent with marked racial predilection, the prevalence varying from about 0.8 per cent in negroids, through 0.2 per cent in Asians to 0.1 per cent or less in white caucasoids. There is no other firm evidence for any other association between high risk of periodontal disease and race. Other genetic diseases that result in defective tissue integrity and host defences and which predispose to periodontal breakdown are, with the exception of Down's syndrome, rare.

Sex. That females are more susceptible to periodontal diseases than males is a commonly held misconception that may have arisen from studies of hospital populations, which are generally biased towards females. Most large surveys now show males to have slightly more severe gingivitis and destructive forms of periodontitis at most ages.

Perinatal events. The early influence of these in establishing a satisfactory immune response may be of importance in explaining the prevalence and severity of some chronic adult diseases. It is not unreasonable to suppose that such events may also affect periodontal diseases although there is, as yet, no definitive evidence for this.

Intercurrent disease. Diabetes mellitus appears to predispose to severe forms of gingivitis and periodontitis; the pathogenesis is probably multifactorial. Severe acquired defects of the immune/inflammatory response (*see* p. 48) certainly produce severe forms of gingivitis and exacerbate periodontal breakdown for a few subjects within a given population. Clinical observation suggests that transient and often trivial intercurrent diseases, such as an attack of gastroenteritis, influenza or even the common cold, may provoke a worsening of gingivitis or a bout of destructive periodontitis. A temporary immune suppression is associated with some infectious diseases, including viral upper respiratory tract infections, and this could adversely imbalance the relationship between subgingival plaque and the host defences.

Drugs. Oral contraceptives, particularly progestogens, enhance gingivitis, and their long-term use may be associated with greater loss of periodontal attachment. By contrast, long-term use of anti-inflammatory drugs, notably non-steroids, may reduce gingivitis in those suffering, for example, from rheumatoid arthritis. However, no significant effects have been demonstrated on the progression of destructive periodontitis.

Diet and nutrition. There is no good evidence that the physical texture of the diet has any influence on periodontal health in man. Apart from severe scurvy (avitaminosis C), no relationship between dietary insufficiency and severe periodontal breakdown has ever been shown conclusively, but a link with subclinical malnutrition is conceivable.

Stress. An association of this with acute necrotizing ulcerative gingivitis (ANUG) has long been recognized and has been suggested for other forms of destructive periodontitis. The influences involved may be similar to those mentioned above for intercurrent disease.

Age. The cumulative effects of past periodontal breakdown obviously increase with age, but susceptibility to periodontal destruction does not worsen. The effect of age on the progression of periodontitis is certainly negligible when good oral hygiene is maintained,[6] and the presence of some plaque, calculus and shallow pocketing is compatible with a functional dentition into old age. However, knowledge of periodontal health and disease in the elderly is meagre because most surveys have been performed in countries with a high prevalence of edentulousness (thought mainly to be the result of other factors). As discussed above, in communities with only limited access to oral health care services, most individuals keep most of their teeth for most of their lives. Treated periodontal patients might appear to be an obvious high-risk group but follow-up studies have shown that they go on to lose few teeth because of periodontal diseases.[7]

Smoking. A number of studies, notably in Scandinavia, show smokers to have generally *higher* levels of plaque and calculus than non-smokers but *less* gingivitis. This paradoxical effect may be due, at least in part, to the peripheral vasoconstriction and impairment of white cell function associated with smoking. However, there is greater loss of alveolar bone in smokers compared to non-smokers, even in those with good oral hygiene. This is likely to be associated with chronically impaired host defences: smoking is, therefore, clearly a risk factor for destructive periodontitis. There is also a higher incidence of ANUG in smokers than in non-smokers.

Markers of susceptibility and activity

Clinical markers. The accuracy, reproducibility and validity of current measurements and indices for periodontal diseases are the source of much discussion. The interpretation of clinical signs has often been wrong in concept, particularly through failure to distinguish between past and present disease activity. Perhaps the best that can be achieved by clinical examination alone is to note the presence of 'severe disease for age'.

Plaque and calculus scores correlate poorly with disease progression. Indices related to *bleeding on probing* have recently become popular but there are indications that their specificity as a predictor of attachment loss is poor. *Bleeding-to-plaque ratios*, particularly when taken repeatedly in a longitudinal study, have some predictive value but, because the events they relate to are transient and superficial, give limited information on true periodontal breakdown. The same can be said for measurements of *gingival crevicular fluid volume* and *flow*. Thus the most common clinical measurements of destructive periodontitis remain *probe-able crevice depth* and *attachment levels*, but these too are fraught with errors and only record disease history.

Do sites with deep pockets or existing loss of attachment really have a greater risk of further breakdown than those with no or little existing destruction? The best answer that can be drawn from the literature is that some 2–3 per cent of sites in patients with a history of moderate to severe periodontal breakdown will experience loss of attachment of more than 2 mm from baseline per year. However, longitudinal studies of this type record a higher percentage of sites with apparently stable or improved attachment levels, so that once again the specificity of the technique is poor.

Haematological and serum markers. Patients with juvenile periodontitis[8] have higher antibody titres to *Actinobacillus actinomycetemcomitans* and to its leucotoxin than either healthy controls or adults with periodontitis, and the titres fall after effective treatment. Similarly, patients with a history of severe adult periodontitis have more IgG antibody to whole cells of *Bacteroides gingivalis* than controls.[9] However, it is not yet clear whether antibody assays can predict a future disease exacerbation.

Markers from saliva. Such markers would be of great value because saliva can be collected non-invasively and highly trained personnel would not be required. If such tests were developed they would have wide application in screening programmes. There is active research in this area, but saliva cannot, of course, provide site-specific information. Disease activity would probably have to be widespread before any putative salivary marker could appear in enough quantity to be detected. Some of the possible future salivary markers of periodontal disease are phenotypic markers of junctional/sulcular epithelium, granulocytes, bacterial enzymes (e.g. trypsin-like activity), elevated IgA/IgG levels and elevated IgA antibodies to *A. actinomycetemcomitans* (for juvenile periodontitis).

Markers from gingival crevicular fluid. This fluid, collected on filter papers placed at the mouth of the crevice for 5–60 seconds, is probably the most promising medium for the detection of disease markers. Collection is technique-sensitive and requires skilled staff, but it is non-invasive and provides site-specific information. Crevicular fluid contains components derived from plasma, from the normal turnover or pathological destruction of host cells, and from bacteria. Lipopolysaccharides (endotoxins) of oral and gingival bacteria have long been implicated as virulence factors in periodontal diseases. The levels of these endotoxins in crevicular fluid correlate with the extent and severity of natural and experimental gingivitis. Many extracellular lytic enzymes are also released by oral micro-organisms, several of which might well degrade gingival and periodontal tissues. Enzyme assay of crevicular fluid is thus attractive as a means of finding such markers, and the recent development of sensitive micro-techniques using fluorescent substrates allows multiple assays to be done at the same time. It has been found that the activity of trypsin-like enzymes correlates with pocket depth, the gingival index and plaque score.

Breakdown products of collagen, such as hydroxyproline, may also prove to be important markers in crevicular fluid. In addition the fluid contains various components of the connective-tissue ground substance: hyaluronic acid in sites with chronic gingivitis and chondroitin 4-sulphate in sites with deep pockets. Chondroitin 4-sulphate, the major glycosaminoglycan (mucopolysaccharide) component of bone, is also found in fluid from sites undergoing orthodontic tooth movement, and may serve as a marker of bone resorption.

Concerning host enzyme markers, levels of collagenase are higher in fluid from sites of periodontitis than from sites with gingivitis only, which in turn have higher levels than healthy crevices. The possibilities of collagenase as a marker of active disease have led to the development of a commercial chairside assay in which paper strips containing crevicular fluid are placed on a collagen-containing gel substrate.[10] Alkaline phosphatase, in high concentration, has also been associated with disease activity, as has beta-glucuronidase.

Specific antibodies against plaque bacteria can be demonstrated in crevicular fluid, and the opsonic activity of these is inversely correlated with gingival health. Cytokines, the 'chemical messengers' that locally regulate several cellular activities including bone resorption, are likely to be involved in periodontal tissue destruction. One such messenger, interleukin-1, can be detected in crevicular fluid. Assays of prostaglandins, which are major mediators of inflammation, hold great promise both as predictors of future disease activity and as indicators of current, site-specific activity. Inhibitors of the enzyme, prostaglandin synthetase, suppress experimental gingivitis in man and significantly inhibit bone loss in experimental animal models of destructive periodontitis. Measurement of prostaglandin E_2 in whole-mouth crevicular fluid has proved sensitive in predicting whether a patient is in remission or about to undergo attachment loss.

Markers from subgingival plaque. Information on the subgingival microflora in health and disease has exploded in the past decade, and over 300 species of micro-organism have so far been identified.[11] There are correlations between the presence in periodontal pockets of substantial numbers of certain putative pathogens and the risk of continuing tissue breakdown, but the fact remains that many individuals can carry these organisms without developing disease. It will therefore take many longitudinal studies before the predictive value of descriptive microbiology can be evaluated fully. The development of gene probes and other rapid diagnostic methods will aid this process.

However, it cannot be over-emphasized that the association of an organism with a diseased periodontal site does not prove a cause-and-effect relationship. Furthermore, the numbers of organisms may bear little relation to their metabolic activity or pathogenic potential – witness the small number of toxic corynibacteria amongst the pharyngeal flora in diptheria. Also, it is the total *activity* of the flora that is relevant, in terms of the cocktail of virulence factors produced and the host response to them. Destructive periodontitis is a mixed infection in which Gram-negative anaerobes appear to be significant and which varies in composition and activity with time. Thus the concept of disease progression being initiated by, or associated with, waves of different microbial consortia in different sites at different times and in different mouths is gaining credence. This makes a taxonomic approach to predicting future disease or indicating current disease activity exceedingly complex and probably unfruitful.

DENTAL CARIES AND ITS RESTORATIVE TREATMENT

(*Sheiham*) The significance of changing patterns has been alluded to in Chapter 2: in most industrialized countries, caries experience has declined by about half in 5-year-olds, 40 per cent in 12-year-olds and by about one-third in 15-year-olds since the early 1970s.[12] Among adults there has been a more modest decline in primary caries and probably a substantial decrease in secondary caries. There may have been a small increase in root caries as more people have retained more teeth for longer.

The changes in the patterns of caries distribution are both in the sites affected and in the rates of progress of established lesions. Thus:

–   The proportion of approximal, buccal and lingual surfaces affected by caries has fallen rapidly as the prevalence of the disease has decreased. Indeed, at the current levels of caries prevalence in most industrialized countries, occlusal lesions constitute the predominant type.

–   The progress of approximal lesions in enamel is generally very slow, and has become even slower in the past 15 years; in addition, fewer enamel lesions are progressing at all (*see* p. 28).

(*Johnson*) There are, however, some countries (for example Iceland) in which caries in children remains very common and is by no means showing a dramatic decline. It is also clear that in all Western communities that have been adequately surveyed, the distribution of caries experience in the population is highly skewed – with a minority of individuals experiencing most of the caries. For instance, in 1986 among 13- and 14-year-olds in the county of Avon, England, a mere 5 per cent had more than half of the affected surfaces and 10 per cent had three-quarters of the approximal lesions; a similar distribution has been found by other investigators.[13] It may be dangerous to assume that the decline in dental caries in Western countries will necessarily continue; indeed, recent data from the London Borough of Camden, an inner city area with some zones of marked social and economic deprivation, show that the proportion of young children with rampant caries is now rising.

As already outlined, statistics in the World Health Organization Global Oral Data Bank suggest that in many developing countries caries prevalence is rising rapidly, with these rising levels crossing over the down-turning graph of some Western countries (Figure facing p. 1).

Shortcomings of restorative treatment

(Elderton) Restorative dentistry can be very effective in improving function and aesthetics, and without restoration many teeth that are saved would be lost prematurely. However, restorative dentistry suffers from a number of failure characteristics.[14] Restorative materials are themselves imperfect, the clinical skills and motivation necessary for their optimum use are often lacking, and objective assessments of restorations indicate that a large proportion are mediocre and contain built-in obsolescence factors. Yet many dentists are quick off the mark to replace restorations that they judge to be imperfect in some way, even though they are frequently unable to state the cause of the problem. Thus it is not unusual for the original errors that caused the 'failure' of the filling to be repeated in the new one, while in the process the cavity increases in size. At each replacement the tooth becomes weaker and the restoration more complex and costly – the 'repeat restoration cycle'.

Superimposed on this is the fact that the presence of caries is often difficult to determine with certainty, and its extent and activity can often only be guessed at. This essential diagnostic problem, together with the very different backgrounds and experiences of individual dentists, make it hardly surprising that diagnosis is found to be very variable and restorative decisions often seem to be idiosyncratic.

People don't 'like' having their teeth filled, yet many patients and dentists appear to believe that restorations are unavoidable. Further, patients who have had many restorations are at particular risk of having many more, for their chances of a dentist finding a need to replace a restoration are higher. Thus, their involvement in a repeat restoration cycle is especially likely, a situation which is fuelled by changing dentist from time to time. The cure for caries lies in changing lifestyles and treatment with fluoride: restorations *per se* do not offer these and hence they do not provide the cure they are often naively believed to effect.

Establishing criteria for restorative treatment

(Anusavice) Decisions on preventive versus restorative treatment are complicated by a lack of well-controlled clinical studies that might indicate the relative effectiveness of these options for preserving the sound hard tissues adjacent to caries or 'defective restorations'. Studies concerning the performance of restorations, or of preventive approaches, have chiefly evaluated marginal integrity and the longevity of materials. They have generally failed to assess the caries risk of individual patients and their findings have often been made under nearly ideal clinical conditions, which may not pertain in private practice throughout the world. In an attempt to improve assessment of the quality and longevity of restorations, an international symposium

Criteria for Placement and Replacement of Dental Restorations was held in Florida in 1987.[15] Two of the important issues discussed are now considered in detail – marginal gaps and caries control.

It is clear that the width of any *marginal gap* in an occlusal restoration is a relatively poor predictor of recurrent caries. Most recurrent lesions associated with extensive amalgam restorations are approximal (on opposing tooth surfaces in the same dental arch), where marginal gaps are difficult to examine. Furthermore, recurrent caries is a major perceived cause of failure of amalgam and composite restorations, confirming that these types of restoration do not cure caries. Little information is available on the rates of caries progression under existing restorations.

Concerning *caries control* and *risk*, the summary from the symposium included the statement:

It was believed that dental caries could be treated away with restorations. This is clearly not the case. Direct filling materials are not as durable as believed by patients and dentists. Furthermore, most materials which are used for dental restorations are associated with initial leakage along the tooth–restoration interface.

Clearly, then it is logical to establish caries control measures as the first step towards restorative treatment, especially for those patients who are considered as above average for, or at high risk of, caries progression. Indeed, the level of risk is most important in assessing the appropriateness of restorative therapy, just as it is in relation to periodontal diseases (*see* p. 17). Numerous well-known factors, such as age, diet, oral hygiene, fluoride exposure and salivary flow rate, are indicators of caries risk, but an overall standard method for risk analysis has not been devised. Because of this, low-risk patients often receive treatment similar to that of high-risk ones. In fact, patients in a low-risk category can inadvertently be shifted towards higher risk for replacement restorations once a first restoration has been placed in a tooth. This is because the majority of restorations are replacements and the criteria for diagnosing caries around restorations are not well defined.

(Johnson) Methods currently used to identify high-risk groups are based on demographic factors, on clinical estimation of past caries experience, on dietary analysis, on the form and arrangement of the teeth, and on laboratory tests performed on samples of saliva, plaque or tooth substance. Commercial kits for chairside testing are now widely available – notably tests for salivary buffering capacity and for the enumeration of *mutans* streptococci and lactobaccilli in saliva.

The usefulness of commercial kits in patient motivation has been argued; some evidence *(Davenport, Hardie, Smith)* is also now emerging for the predictive value of such bacteriological tests. For example, salivary *Streptococcus mutans* and lactobacillus levels were found to have some relationship to caries activity when saliva collected from 93 six-year-old children was assayed, and the tests repeated on 73 of these children a year later. The mean index of decayed, missing and filled surfaces of the eight deciduous molars had increased from 2.3 at the initial examination to 3.5; the mean salivary *S. mutans* levels showed a corresponding but not statistically significant increase over the same period, but there were positive correlations between the index scores at the second examination and the salivary *mutans* and lactobacillus levels found at the initial visit.

(Anusavice) Overall does the existing scientific evidence provide better means of establishing criteria for restorative treatment than the traditional, operational approach? Certainly, there are specific issues that have not yet been resolved scientifically. For example:

- The relative rate of activity or progression of caries adjacent to restorations as a function of risk factors (diet, bacteria, oral hygiene, etc.) has not been determined from a well-designed clinical study.

- The quality of replacement restorations compared with the quality of the original restoration has not been extensively evaluated.

- The characteristics of micro-organisms in marginal gap regions within restored teeth have not yet been established.

(Foster) Although secondary caries is the major reason given for the replacement of restorations, its diagnosis and the consequent treatment decisions are extremely variable.[16] In this context, the relationship between the acidogenic ratio of plaque from the margins of defective amalgam restorations and that of generalized plaque in the same individual could serve as a method of predicting the presence of 'active' secondary caries around dubiously defective margins. To examine this, 80 patients with amalgam restorations having defective margins each had a plaque sample taken from such margins and another from smooth tooth surfaces. The ratio of acidogenic to total organisms was then calculated for both sites. A large difference between the two acidogenic ratios was predictive of active caries in the majority of cases. However, a small difference successfully predicted the absence of caries in only just over half of cases. As yet it appears that the sensitivity of this method did not improve upon the initial diagnosis made by routine clinical means.

Prevention and the bitewing radiograph

(Pitts) Traditionally, bitewing radiographs have been an aid to dental examinations, detecting small carious lesions (in particular those on approximal surfaces) not evident by clinical means alone. In most cases, once a lesion had been detected by this means, the decision to restore was almost 'automatic'. However, as detailed below, great emphasis is now being placed on the need to preserve tooth tissue and to avoid invasive treatment wherever

possible. Also, rather than being regarded as an inherent weakness, truly arrested lesions are now seen as more resistant to future carious attack than sound enamel.

For patients who can be expected or persuaded to return for review appointments, the current philosophy is that smaller approximal radiolucencies (those radiographically confined to the enamel and, in certain cases, to the outer dentine) should *not* be immediately or indiscriminately restored, but should be treated preventively and reviewed after an interval appropriate to the individual patient. Some lesions, including more advanced ones, may already have become arrested by the time the dentist first identifies them, so the size of the lesion *per se* cannot serve as the sole criterion dictating the need for a restoration. However, for lesions where there is no evidence of arrest, it would be very useful to have an agreed restorative threshold based upon radiographic appearance.

(Anusavice) Smooth surface lesions that have not penetrated the enamel–dentine junction should certainly be treated with a preventive 'package' including topical fluoride. Patients should also be taught that, with proper hygiene on their part, it is possible to arrest and even remineralize these lesions. Indeed, all concerned need to appreciate that only when caries has penetrated well into dentine should operative intervention be considered – but just because a lesion has penetrated dentine does not on its own mean that a restoration is inevitable. Preventive measures take time to exert their effect; and lesions not already arrested must be given the chance to do so.

(Pitts) 'Monitoring' by radiography for preventive purposes means that greater attention should be paid to radiation exposure, to standardization of exposure geometry by the use of film holders, and to quality assurance. But the developments described above also demand reappraisal of the rationale for bitewing radiography. Although some progress has been made with other diagnostic methods, such as fibre-optic transillumination, the bitewing technique is still regarded by most authorities as the best method of identifying small lesions (including enamel lesions) on contacting approximal surfaces. However, the replies from 1127 dentists in Scotland to a questionnaire concerning treatment options have demonstrated that there is still considerable scope for persuading many operators to adopt a more positive approach when using bitewings as an aid to caries management. The dentists were asked to indicate the minimum point (threshold) at which they felt a filling should be placed for a 12-year-old patient and for a 30-year-old patient. For the 12-year-old, 43 per cent said they would wait until a radiolucency had reached the dentine, but the majority said they would elect to restore radiolucencies that were confined to the enamel (10 per cent of these wanted to restore small radiolucencies in the outer half of the enamel). The results for the 30-year-old were a little more encouraging, with 70 per cent of the dentists indicating that they would wait for radiographic dentine involve-

ment, although the remainder still elected to restore radiolucencies confined to the enamel.

The predictive accuracy of bitewings

(Benn, Watson) The association between the radiographic appearance of approximal caries and the presence of cavitation appears to have changed dramatically over recent years, at least in some regions with falling caries incidence. In 1970, reported cavitation rates were 34, 66 and 87 per cent for outer enamel, inner enamel and outer dentine radiographic lesions respectively, but by 1986 these figures had fallen to 7, 12 and 51 per cent.[17] This means that accurate radiographic assessment of cavitation and progression has become even more important.

Unfortunately, where unstandardized film positioning is used to measure lesion depth and rates of progression as a guide for preventive or restorative decisions, unreliable data are probably being generated. In a laboratory model the accuracy of bitewing radiographs of approximal caries was considerably affected by the X-ray path through the tooth, the precise effect varying with the depth of the lesion. Thus, when using unstandardized bitewing radiographs, it is unlikely that the true depth of a lesion can be determined accurately from its image because the apparent depth of the feature can be increased or decreased by *small* differences in the beam angle. Indeed, a carious lesion apparently involving dentine on radiographs may be caused by a lesion that is, in reality, confined to the enamel. The implications for the monitoring of lesions in general practice are that:

- Shallow enamel lesions may show on a radiograph but then not appear on a subsequent film if the X-ray path is changed.

- Deeper enamel lesions may falsely project radiographic lesions at some beam orientations and their appearances may alter if that orientation changes between radiographs.

- There is around a 50 per cent chance that even if true outer dentine demineralization has occurred, cavitation will not be present.

Accurate measurements of the extent of demineralization or remineralization cannot be made with beam angle changes of greater than ±3°. However, the apparent radiographic depth of a lesion is, from a clinical standpoint, a less important indicator of carious activity than the rate of progression – and this measurement can only be made accurately from standardized bitewing films. It would seem necessary to standardize the repositioning of the film in the mouth to ±3° from the original position.[18]

(Benn) A repositionable bitewing film holder has been developed and is on clinical trial for use in general dental practice, with the goal of achieving

a repositioning accuracy of ±3° in two planes. It has two broad flat occlusal biting platforms that cross both sides of the dental arch. These stabilize the holder and ensure that the interocclusal space will be in the middle of the film, which is important for monitoring alveolar bone as well as approximal lesions. The holder position is recorded by noting where the anterior edges of the occlusal platforms cross the upper arch on the left and right sides; and three measurements are recorded for each side. In total, about 25 seconds are required to position, record, irradiate and check the film holder position.

Other aspects of caries research

(Watson) Advances are being made on several other research fronts. For example, the histological assessment of carious lesions has generally been undertaken by examining ground sections with ordinary or polarized transmitted light microscopy. The production of thin (under $100 \mu m$ thickness) sections is time-consuming and technically difficult but, with a tandem scanning (confocal) reflected light microscope, intact block faces of specimens can now be examined without thin sectioning. This instrument will produce thin (2–3 μ m), high-resolution images of optical sections below the surface of semi-transparent specimens such as teeth. Sections 1.2 mm thick, with $300 \mu m$ of tissue lost as kerf between the slices, can be examined in the condition left by the saw, without further polishing, and information obtained from both sides of the section $10 \mu m$ below the cut surfaces. Fluorescent staining of carious lesions can further improve the image contrast between mineralized and demineralized tooth tissue.

(Wahab, Shellis) Further work is needed to determine the differential effects of fluoride (*see* p. 30) on both the bacterial and chemical aspects of cariogenesis. In an experimental system *in vitro*, where caries was inhibited partly at 1 part per milion (p.p.m.) F and completely at 2 and 5 p.p.m. F, fluoride did not affect the terminal pH or total acid production but it did slow the rate of pH fall, thus reducing the time spent below the critical pH. Loss of calcium from enamel was greatest at 0 p.p.m. F and much less at 1 and 2 p.p.m. Fluoride was released from the enamel at 0 p.p.m. F but at 1 p.p.m. there was no net change and at 2 p.p.m. there was net uptake. It thus seems that fluoride at 1–5 p.p.m affects lesion formation only partly by affecting bacterial metabolism (slowing down the rate of pH fall); the main effect is through its influence on mineral chemistry.

Advances in caries management

(Lester) A number of responsible and appropriate approaches to caries management have been made in Australia, where there is a widespread

tendency for politicians and health administrators to congratulate their dentists for unprecedented success in health care, but then to query their worldly wisdom in voluntarily removing the major reason for their existence and source of income. It is relevant, therefore, to examine the current practice of caries prevention and management for the population in terms of the future and well-being of the profession in general and of its restorative arm in particular.

Undoubtedly, the initiation and maintenance of artificially fluoridated water supplies to some two-thirds of all Australians is *the* major advance in caries management over the last 20 years. Together with other forms of fluoride delivery, including fluoride supplements and fluoridated toothpaste, and in the presence of improved oral hygiene, the result has been a huge fall in the mean number of decayed, missing and filled teeth from over 8 to 1.8 for 12-year-old children. A mean of 1.5 is confidently predicted for this age group by 1991.[19] Studies elsewhere also continue to confirm the value of fluoridated water, but it is important that a substantially decreased caries incidence is also being recorded in non-fluoridated areas in Australia.[20]

It is as well to remember that the fluoride ion increases caries resistance by a variety of mechanisms including:

— increased insolubility of the enamel in acid;

— increased rate of post-eruptive enamel maturation;

— inhibition of plaque formation and acid production;

— remineralization of early carious lesions;

— improved tooth morphology expressed as shallower fissures.

The residual problem

As with most developed countries, there is little doubt then that the acute caries 'epidemic' in Australia has largely been eradicated. But success or failure is always relative, and while caries experience in children and adolescents has greatly decreased, it is likely that a plateau will soon be reached. There is also, as in other countries (*see* p. 23), an increasing awareness that a small proportion of the younger population has a very high caries experience. The burden of care created by caries, while no longer overwhelming, is still a sizeable problem in the adolescent population. It thus seems that a considerable level of need for restorative services will remain among children and adolescents, though concentrated in an 'at risk' group which, despite much research, is not yet easily identifiable.

The earlier victims of the caries 'epidemic', with the amalgam defence mounted against it, are now in adulthood coping with the well-known problems of multiple surface, oft-replaced restorations and the fragility of the remaining tooth structure. A pertinent question now is: 'Is restoration management succeeding or failing?' Some light is thrown on this matter by the process of peer review.

Peer review and quality assurance

The principles underlying these methods insist that efforts be made to analyse in a rational way the outcome of patient-related activities. For instance, occasional examples of gross over-treatment have been brought out by an internal search at one Australian dental school. A single example will suffice. A patient came for *routine* assessment and treatment and with no particular problems from his point of view. After 65 active treatments, the patient is still under care, still with 'appalling' oral hygiene, and with partial denture castings waiting for try-in because he is temporarily away. When he returns, the castings are unlikely to be of any use.

This sort of anomaly can perhaps be explained by the fact that young, recently graduated staff look for 'things to do' and pieces of metal or plastic to place, instead of being inclined to more rational, integrated care. These staff have been educated in the clinic as undergraduates using an itemized system where certain numbers of each kind of various treatments were required to obtain an assessment of progress. This approach has now been discontinued in the final year at the particular school, in line with changes at other schools around the world.

For dentists employed in hospitals, evidence of continuing peer review is a requirement for accreditation established by the Australian Council of Hospital Standards. However, the application of quality assurance to private dentistry remains a challenge for the future; the threat of legal action against the surveying body appears to be the main reason for it not having been embraced whole-heartedly by the local Dental Associations. The process promises much and would be a real sign of the profession's maturity and self-confidence.

The anti-amalgam debate

This flared up recently in Australia as a result of an article published in a popular and reputable consumer magazine expressing concern over the safety of the mercury content of amalgam restorations. The article suggested that if a composite resin was to be recommended as strong enough for '...your next filling, you have more than a cosmetic reason to choose it'. However, the scientific evidence is under continual review and a recent official report,[21] while drawing attention to the hazards of persistent occupational exposure to mercury, concludes:

There is no documented scientific evidence to show adverse effects from mercury in dental amalgam restorations, except in rare cases of mercury hypersensitivity, and on present evidence the routine use of composite as an amalgam substitute cannot be endorsed.

Amalgam restorations and the reasons for and effects of their replacement have also been under review in a more clinical, operative sense. The figure (from Scotland) of 50 per cent survival at five years after placement[22] is an obvious cause for concern, whether it be the fault of the material, the operator or the patient.

Non-invasive management of caries

This approach requires some fundamental re-thinking of concepts by those already trained in an essentially restorative attitude to caries management.

Heavy metal fluoride. The following is largely an account of the present approach in the Sydney Faculty Department of Preventive Dentistry, which has been developed out of a concern to decrease unnecessary physical and emotional damage to children in the name of dental health.

Three levels of clinical circumstance determine three clinical regimens for the topical application of fluoride agents:

— Free smooth (buccal and lingual) tooth surfaces with early caries, and sound smooth surfaces prior to orthodontic banding: 10 per cent stannous fluoride solution is applied to the cleaned and dried teeth for four minutes. (Note: 2 per cent sodium fluoride is the agent of choice when bands are in place.)

— Newly erupted teeth, susceptible pits and fissures before the teeth have erupted sufficiently to allow sealing, and early enamel lesions on approximal surfaces of posterior teeth: a 10 per cent stannous fluoride paste is applied to the cleaned, dried teeth and covered with a 'bandage' (Stomahesive or Varihesive wafer), which subsequently dissolves in the oral fluids.[23]

— Advanced enamel lesions in all surfaces of posterior teeth, dentine lesions in posterior teeth to be controlled chemically, and 'sticky' fissures (to provide a prolonged fluoride treatment at a separate visit before fissure sealing): silver fluoride is applied for three minutes followed by 10 per cent stannous fluoride paste placed under a Stomahesive wafer. A week or two later the process may be repeated, or the tooth is sealed or restored (described below).

This approach certainly has its proponents but the strategies do not always meet with universal (or national) favour, concerns being expressed in some quarters about safety (possible soft-tissue trauma and ingestion); specificity (the application of solution to all available surfaces); the possibility of discoloration in teeth and existing restorations; and, in some cases, efficacy (the incompleteness of data on effectiveness).

Fissure sealant. In the Sydney scheme, pit and fissure sealants for the primary prevention of caries in sound untreated teeth are recommended at 3–4 years of age for first and second deciduous molars; 6–7 years for first permanent molars; and 11–13 years for second permanent molars. No specific recommendations are made for premolars. Simonsen[24] has found that 60 per cent of sealants are retained over a 10-year period and now recommends an unfilled, autopolymerizing, white composite resin.

Placement of sealant over questionable or incipient caries in occlusal fissures has been recommended after careful consideration of the available evidence.[25] In essence this alters the local environment through an immediate and major reduction in the bacterial count from acid etching, by preventing entry of nutrients into the fissure, and by a continuing reduction in viability of the remaining bacteria. The approach is cost-effective, painless and conservative of tooth structure, but meticulous attention to technique is required. The Australian experience that approximately three-quarters of decayed or restored sites in 12-year-olds are associated with pits and fissures emphasizes the potential preventive value of this approach.

There is room for debate as to whether there should be selectivity in sealant use, based upon the child's caries experience. *(Martens)* Each situation requires individual consideration, although a complete preventive programme involving dietary management, good hygiene and daily use of fluoride is essential. It is difficult to propose general rules for the application of pit and fissure sealants, but many feel that their use should certainly not be *carte blanche*; rather, they are only indicated for teeth with initial lesions in the fissure regions. In addition, however, sealants may be especially appropriate for apparently sound teeth in certain special 'at risk' patients, including the mentally retarded and physically handicapped who cannot brush adequately, those treated under general anaesthesia, and those with occlusal surface abnormalities or additional pits and grooves due to developmental disturbances (e.g. fusion or gemination).

Invasive management of caries in deciduous teeth

(Lester) Craig and co-workers[26] have promoted an 'atraumatic' approach on the premise that carious deciduous teeth have a finite life span, and that different rules therefore apply than for permanent teeth, such that simpler treatment will suffice. Time may be bought, by this means, for the child to develop into a more mature, easily treated and less sensitive patient. They advocate the avoidance of injections and matrix bands, the minimal use of high-speed handpieces and high-volume suction and, instead, the use of sharp

excavators for caries removal and cotton-roll clamps for lower arch isolation. This is very difficult ground in a philosophical, even emotional, sense but worthy of careful consideration and further analysis of the clinical data.

After the topical application of silver fluoride followed by stannous fluoride paste and a Stomahesive wafer (*see* list above), there may be an open cavity for restoration. When this is the case, the cavity floor is checked after 1–2 weeks to ensure a black matt appearance before restoration with *glass-ionomer cement*. These cements have many applications in the restorative treatment of deciduous teeth with their relatively light masticatory loading. Chemical bonding, fluoride release, aesthetics, reduced cavity preparation and correspondingly less need for analgesia are all advantages of these materials. For approximal lesions in deciduous molars a 'slot' preparation only is required, except for distal surface lesions in first molars where an occlusal 'lock' is needed. Syringe placement of the material with no matrix band is the norm, as cavity extension is minimal and there is no packing force to contend with. The material can be contoured while plastic and then carved. The marginal ridge should be rounded as the material has a low edge strength.

Preventive restorations

(*Anusavice*) As implied above, before any invasive restorative therapy is started, repeated attempts must be made to shift the patient from a high to a lower caries risk category, after which a more conservative treatment plan may be considered. Coupled to this objective is the need to think about alternatives to the materials and techniques that are widely, if sometimes incorrectly, assumed to require the removal of large amounts of sound dental hard tissue in order to establish an 'ideal' outline form (cavity shape). When operative intervention is indicated, the position, size, and shape of the cavity preparation should be based primarily on the extent of the lesion rather than upon a traditional or preconceived 'outline form'.[27] Pit and fissure sites with small lesions, or where the activity of a lesion is in doubt, should be managed by sealant rather than by tooth cutting and filling. For larger cavities in high-stress areas, an amalgam restoration may be placed, although research with certain posterior composites suggests that these should sometimes be used instead; marginal leakage may be virtually eliminated adjacent to composite restorations in which the margins are confined entirely to enamel.

The composites come into their own in posterior teeth when the *preventive resin* restoration technique is used, whereby the overtly carious part of the surface of a tooth is restored and the remaining fissures are sealed. Referred to in the UK as the *sealant restoration*, the preventive resin restoration forms a bridge between non-invasive and invasive techniques for the treatment of caries in fissured surfaces. (*Lester*) It is a truly conservative technique which is tooth-coloured, mercury-free and easy to repair. This is an extremely

important concept in furthering an understanding of 'quality' in tooth preparation and restoration. At recall there can be little temptation to replace
the restored area or areas if the sealant part remains intact; and a partially
debonded sealant can be economically and conservatively corrected with an
acid-etch procedure and further sealant.

Light-cured composite materials

(Crocker) It is pertinent here to reflect upon the fact that the part of dentistry
concerned with fillings, crowns and bridges is known, in some parts of the
world, as conservative dentistry, yet it is only with the advent of adhesive
restorative materials that the term has become justifiable. Cutting can now
largely be restricted to the removal of diseased tooth tissue, especially when
materials are used that are adhesive to dentine as well as to enamel. Some
simple guidelines to increase the likelihood of success are as follows.

—   Institute good plaque control before doing permanent restorative
    work.

—   If etched enamel is required, then apply knowledge of tooth micro-
    morphology to ensure that the ends of enamel prisms will be exposed
    to the acid. Bevel the enamel only if this is needed to expose prisms
    ends.

—   Before any material is used, read all the instructions; even better, find
    out the theory behind the instructions.

—   Leave enough time, especially for occlusal adjustments. A rushed job
    where each stage is not given full time is better not done at all.

—   Composite materials should be placed in very small increments, even
    if a powerful curing light is used. If this is not done, the stresses created
    in the tooth can be immense, as can the internal stresses in the
    material itself. These may lead to premature breakdown of the resto-
    ration by chewing forces and/or by solvents and oils in food.

—   Make sure that there is no water contamination; use of rubber dam
    conforms with excellent practice.

—   Cracking of teeth after the placement of large amalgams bounded on
    both sides by enamel is an important reason for adopting, where
    possible, an alternative type of restoration.

—   Composite incisal edge restorations and porcelain veneers are much
    more conservative than crowns and should be used in preference
    where possible.

— Think of ways of being a real conservationist. Never destroy tooth structure if this can be avoided.

The tunnel restoration

(Lester) This has been promoted by Knight[28] and others, applying the inherent physical and chemical advantages of glass-ionomer cement to posterior approximal lesions where there is an intact marginal ridge to be retained. The preparation requires minimal removal of sound tooth structure, so reducing the likelihood of future fracture of associated cusps. Because glass-ionomer cement bonds to both prepared enamel and dentine, the total removal of weakened enamel and the provision of undercuts are unnecessary. The recent introduction of the radiopaque ionomer cement (cermet) has overcome what have been seen as some of the disadvantages of the technique. The major problems experienced clinically are how adequately to remove caries in the contact area without damaging the adjacent tooth and uncertainties concerning the removal of fractured enamel.

Bonded bridgework

It stands to reason that dentists should be particularly discerning when it comes to using the more extensive adhesive-retained restorations such as fixed bridges. *(Aboush)* Various restorations may be present in the abutment teeth of resin-bonded bridgework and clinicians need to know the extent to which retainers will bond to these. With this in mind, the bond strengths of an adhesive resin cement (Panavia) to etched enamel, composite resin and amalgam, and to adherends consisting of 50 per cent etched enamel and 50 per cent restorative material, have been measured. The mean tensile bond strengths, in MPa were: enamel 28, composite resin 25, amalgam 8, enamel/composite 21, enamel/amalgam 6, which suggests that bonding with the resin cement to unfavourable components of restored teeth should be avoided where possible. In a further study, the tensile bond strengths of both thick (bulk) and thin films of three resin cements (Adhesive Bridge Cement, Panavia and Super-Bond) to a Ni–Cr alloy (Wiron 88) were compared. With all the cements, values for thin-film specimens were significantly higher than those for thick specimens, indicating the need for accurately fitting resin-bonded bridges.

The restorative scene changes continually and new developments should be critically examined as and when they occur. *(Howden)* A new concept in bridgework recently introduced in a number of countries involves titanium attachments (Universal Dental Attachments®, Ambitec S.A. and Dokon Attachments®, Medicon S.A) which are fixed to abutment teeth with pins and adhesives. Tooth preparation is thereby confined to the discing of facets on the mesial or distal aspects of the abutments and the cutting of two to four pinholes, 2.1 mm long, into these surfaces using a template and special drill. The attachments are then fixed and impressions taken for the laboratory construction of a pontic. The necessary laboratory expertise is, however, limited as 'copings' are available to facilitate construction of the metal framework. Alternatively, a pontic covered with self-curing acrylic can be fabricated at the chairside. Pins can be inserted into previously prepared cavities filled with posterior composite resin or into suitable crowns already present on the abutment teeth. The concept of 'immediate' tooth replacement has thus become a possibility at a lower cost than for conventional or for some types of resin-bonded bridgework.

DENTAL DISEASE AND THE DENTATE ELDERLY

Reference has already been made to the increasing numbers of elderly dentate people throughout the world. *(Hall Dexter)* As the regularly attending patient grows older the dangers of 'supervised neglect' may increase. Over a period of years problems may develop that cannot be discovered at a brief recall appointment. This raises the issues of how frequently full radiographic assessments should be made and what systems and frequency of periodontal examination and monitoring should be followed. If the periodontal condition of an ageing person becomes unstable, how much more quickly does attachment loss and loss of supporting bone occur than in a younger patient? These questions are asked in the certain clinical experience that a patient who has appeared stable for years may suddenly undergo rapid alveolar bone loss at one or more sites within a period of months. Some, albeit incomplete, answers are provided in the above section on periodontal diseases. The fundamental question is whether the objective of 'teeth for life' is desirable in each and every case (*see* p. 16); some susceptible individuals, who will only keep destructive periodontal disease at bay by maintaining a very high standard of plaque control, find this an increasingly difficult burden as old age approaches.

Multiple restorations also create considerable problems and recurrent caries may not be at all easy to identify. Pulps may unobtrusively die, without pain, under large restorations. So, how much emphasis should be placed upon routine pulp vitality testing? And how often should root-filled teeth be radiographed? Similar sentiments apply to the 'cracked tooth' syndrome. How thoroughly and frequently should diagnostic procedures be carried out to check for teeth with cracks propagating through the dentine; and at what stage is restorative intervention indicated as a preventive measure to avoid a tooth splitting? Then, in an increasing number of individuals, there is a continuing loss of dental hard tissues from the effects of attrition, abrasion or erosion and, in many cases, a combination of these factors. The decision as to when to intervene with restorative/reconstructive dentistry is extremely difficult.

It may be that the essential answer to most of these questions is 'use your clinical experience' – but this is a totally unsatisfactory solution in an age of scientifically-based care and at a time of increasing accountability. And young members of the profession do not possess 'experience', while the older ones may apply yesterday's criteria (see p. 10). There is, of course, a need to improve the motivation of the elderly dentate toward preserving their dentitions and, in this context, *(Kluter, Plasschaert, Truin, Wimmers)* preventive self-care packages, comprising oral hygiene instruction, oral hygiene aids and a teaching manual for dentate subjects aged 55–75 years are being evaluated in the Netherlands.

Root caries

(Lester) Root caries is an increasing problem, especially as patients retain their teeth for longer and undergo gingival recession. Development of the lesion requires the exposure of the root surface to the oral environment – and the subsequent colonization of this surface by plaque, probably of a different nature to that associated with coronal caries. The causes relate generally to altered health status, lifestyle and diet, nutrition, salivary flow, and loss of manual dexterity.

Where there is root caries, oral hygiene routines should be upgraded and broad-spectrum antimicrobial mouthwashes (especially 0.2 per cent chlorhexidine) and topical fluoride applications should be instituted. The least severe lesions can usually be controlled in this way, and sometimes advanced ones also. Smoothing and polishing (in conjunction with topical fluoride) are sometimes recommended and, where access allows, lesions may be restored with glass-ionomer cement alone or in conjunction with composite resin in a 'sandwich technique'. Overall, attempting to bring about arrest of all these lesions makes a great deal of sense and this may prove to be the choice method of management, with restorations being used in addition solely for appearance or functional purposes.

Dentures

The need for complete dentures should, of course, be avoided at all costs. *(Ksiazkiewicz-Jozwiak)* Loss of teeth causes disturbances of many functions of the stomatognathic system, including speech. Dentures affect vocal tract geometry by changing the way in which the mouth functions as a sound resonator; they also affect the function of the tongue, lips and cheeks. Lisp, hiss and whizz are the most frequent speech disturbances in patients with complete dentures, and the positioning of the anterior teeth plays an important part in speech rehabilitation. When this positioning and the degree of speech deformation are investigated with three-dimensional sound recordings (sonograms), clear relationships can be found between lower anterior tooth position and pronunciation. In particular, the distinctiveness of pronunciation is more related to the posterior teeth. A period of adaptation to the prostheses has a positive influence on speech distinctiveness.

ORTHODONTICS

(Tala) Orthodontics became a specialty of dentistry at the end of last century. It has grown considerably, so that in Denmark, for example, it absorbs a considerable proportion (32 per cent) of all oral health resources. In Finland the number of children receiving orthodontic care in the public sector has increased from 7000 in 1972 to almost 100 000 in 1985, and public health administrators have expressed their concern regarding this expansion.

Orthodontic care has special features that make it different from many other areas of dentistry. Treatment usually takes a long time, often several years, and demand usually far exceeds supply. Consequently the cost of treatment per patient is high. From the public health viewpoint, this amounts to a heavy burden loaded into a health care system with thousands of other needs and challenges. Private orthodontics, operating on the principle of demand and supply, is, of course, usually outside public control.

(Shaw) The availability, organization, and financing of orthodontic services naturally have an important bearing on the uptake of treatment. The capacity for orthodontics in any dental system reflects the number of dentists who undertake some orthodontics, the proportion who are in full-time specialist orthodontic practice, whether or not they employ auxiliaries, and the number of patients a single orthodontist is able to treat. This number is also the main determinant of treatment standards. When all barriers to receiving orthodontic care are removed, the uptake of treatment may be as high as 60 per cent; in other words, children who do not receive treatment become a minority.

The funding of orthodontic services is also remarkably different from one country to the next, and in some the family must meet the entire cost of treatment. More commonly, treatment is either free or partly funded by state or private insurances that reimburse the user, often in proportion to the degree of severity of malocclusion as assessed by some form of treatment priority index (*see* next section). Thus, for children with minor dental irregularities or those living in a setting of purely private orthodontics, uptake of treatment will simply reflect an ability and willingness to pay. Priority indexing, such as in Sweden, is intended to aid in the distribution of resources so that the treatment remains of a high standard, and to protect children from unnecessary treatment of acceptable malocclusions.

Levels of prescription of medical and dental care are known to be strongly influenced by the system of remuneration. In orthodontics, payment systems that calculate fees on the number of appliance components have encouraged the use of multiple appliances; low fees in general promote large case-loads, while low fixed-appliance fees encourage over-prescription of treatment with removable appliances.

The need for orthodontic treatment

(Tala) The perceived extent of dentofacial anomalies and orthodontic treatment needs varies widely because of the inherent subjectivity involved. In most World Health Organization pathfinder surveys, the proportion of 12-year-olds with malocclusions has been around 10 per cent. The 1982 nationwide report from the Finnish communal health centres revealed that 15 per cent of parents considered their 7–16-year-old children to be in need of orthodontic treatment, whereas the health centre dentists found this to be so for 18 per cent. Both parents and dentists were in agreement in 84 per cent of the cases.

The World Health Organization manual on oral health surveys[29] distinguishes two levels of occlusal anomaly (aside from gross defects) as follows:

- slight anomalies, such as one or more rotated or tilted teeth or slight crowding or spacing which disturb the regular alignment of the teeth;

- more serious anomalies, specifically, the presence of one or more of the following conditions of the incisors: maxillary overjet of 9 mm or more, mandibular overjet, anterior crossbite equal to or greater than a full tooth depth, open bite, a midline shift greater than 4 mm, and crowding or spacing estimated to be greater than 4 mm.

The central problem is to define the malocclusions for which treatment is justified on health grounds and which should therefore be treated by the public health care system. Also to be taken into consideration, of course, are the desires and aspirations of patients and parents.

Several indices have been developed to estimate the prevalence and severity of dentofacial anomalies, though most have been unhelpful in defining who should be treated. The socio-psychological aspects of malocclusion, though important, are almost impossible to estimate objectively. There is therefore little doubt that orthodontic treatment provision is dependent upon subjective judgements by professionals and by the equally subjective desire of patients and their parents. In addition, orthodontic treatment needs are sometimes simply induced by dentists.

(Shaw) The need for clear, well-founded risk–benefit appraisal is over-

whelming and the orthodontic profession has an urgent ethical responsibility to develop this. The time appears to have come for the profession to consider, rather more universally, the use of some objective form of index of treatment need. Certainly in this age of increasing accountability, orthodontics is attracting the attention of health economists working on behalf of socialized services or insurance schemes.

A general way to determine the level of individual treatment need is by an index with dental health and aesthetic components.[30] While a major shortcoming of any indexing system is the risk of insensitivity and misjudgement of individual needs, obvious advantages include uniformity among practitioners and safeguards for the patient, opportunities for patient counselling, and for resource allocation and planning.

(Tala) The 1979 World Health Organization guide to oral health epidemiological investigations,[31] in listing the indications for orthodontic treatment, took into account traits that may predispose to increased risk of:

— tooth loss from caries, periodontal diseases, trauma or root resorption;

— physiological disturbances of function (mandibular joint disorders, speech defects or masticatory disturbances);

— socio-psychological disturbances.

(Shaw) Traditionally orthodontists have assumed a mainly utilitarian motive for their work – that orthodontic treatment enhances dental health and function, and as such assures greater longevity of the dentition. There is, however, a disappointing lack of evidence for these aspirations and the disadvantages of malocclusion from the dental health and functional viewpoint appear rather modest. Early correction of prominent incisors certainly may reduce the risk of trauma: the potential benefit becomes less with age but it should not be forgotten that there is also some association between excessive overjet and pathological migration of the incisors in adulthood. Avoidance of pathological changes that may attend tooth impaction (especially of wisdom teeth) is clearly desirable. Of other variations in alignment, only the extreme, such as deep overbite and gross displacement of individual teeth, are likely to be true risks to dental health. Links between most occlusal variations and dental caries, periodontal disease and mandibular dysfunction are weak, so that in recent years greater emphasis has been placed upon the role of orthodontics in enhancing social and psychological well-being through improvement in appearance.

While conspicuous dental defects may attract childhood teasing, facial attractiveness is, in general, apparently more salient than dental appearance, such that the social response to many minor dental irregularities seems to be insignificant. The extent of individual adjustment to unsightly malocclusion varies considerably, ranging from deep concern to complete disregard. Those with a conspicuous malocclusion will often, even without treatment, continue to make their way through life as well adjusted and accomplished as others around them, with little impairment of their quality of life. However, dissatisfaction with dental appearance felt in childhood may remain for a lifetime, so the individual need for orthodontic treatment should be judged with some sensitivity.

Risks associated with orthodontic treatment

As with most medical and paramedical intervention, orthodontic treatment is not without risks. A small but permanent loss of periodontal attachment may occur with tooth movement in a significant number of individuals even when standards of oral hygiene are high, although a group of patients who had received fixed appliance treatment 35 years before had no more (or less) periodontal disease than a matched control group.[32] Even so, root resorption, which may be severe, is common with fixed appliances, and all appliances may predispose to an increased susceptibility to caries. Orthodontic treatment may also lead to occlusal dysfunction, despite the fact that elimination of occlusal disturbances is one of its aims and benefits. This is an ironic possibility, the risk of which appears to be less with fixed than with removable appliance therapy. Not uncommonly an excessive and occasionally traumatic overbite is created by treatment, particularly with removable appliances where overbite control during the treatment of prominent upper incisors has been inadequate. In addition to these factors, there may, of course, be some degree of failure in meeting the planned goals of treatment.

Indeed, perhaps the greatest risk in orthodontic treatment is that of partial or total failure to accomplish a worthwhile, lasting change. Follow-up surveys of North American patients allow some generalizations to be made: overbites reduced during edgewise treatment tend to increase later; mandibular intercanine expansion tends to relapse; a degree of crowding tends to return; and the lower incisor region tends to develop late crowding, almost regardless of previous extractions and alignment.

(Tala) Another interesting evaluation of the long-term results of orthodontic care has recently been made in Sweden. All 3000 'completed' orthodontic cases from 1976–86 at the University of Malmo were considered. Sixty-three per cent of the treatments were deemed successful and 8 per cent had failed, while the remaining 29 per cent never received the treatment or it was interrupted. In only half the cases did the treatment result in so-called normal occlusion. Overall, the quality of the orthodontic care was considered to be good; failures were usually due to lack of co-operation and/or to wrong diagnosis and prognosis. It was held indisputable that children with severe malocclusions should be treated and that this was a reasonable call upon public health care funds. However, where the dentofacial anomaly was slight,

it was felt that the subjective need for treatment should be investigated in depth so that only those with high motivation would be included in the treatment programme, and that treatment should then be at the patient's/parents' own expense.

(Shaw) In a stringent review of Norwegian patients treated mainly with fixed appliances, only 43 per cent of treatments were regarded as fully successful. The majority may have gained substantial improvement, but it must be said that such an outcome would be less likely where removable appliances are used more widely. Indeed, in such a group treated in Britain, only 29 per cent were found to have improved substantially, as judged by a numerical index of tooth alignment.[33] Naturally, a crucial factor in the success of orthodontic treatment is patient co-operation. In fixed appliance therapy, non-compliance in the use of elastics or headgear commonly leads to anchorage loss. With removable appliances, the biggest problem is, of course, not wearing the appliance, and disturbingly high discontinuation rates occur among British patients.

The available evidence suggests that the balance between risk and benefit in orthodontics is delicate. In general terms, the patient has the best chance of gaining an overall benefit when the original malocclusion is severe and the treatment is delivered expertly. Conversely, the patient has the best chance of not benefitting, or indeed of sustaining an overall loss, when the original malocclusion is mild, and inexpert or perfunctory treatment is provided. This does not, of course, mean that non-specialist practitioners have no part to play (*see* Chapter 5). Rather, they have a significant role in the early detection of malocclusion, in the wise and, if necessary, interceptive management of the developing dentition, and in undertaking tooth movements commensurate with their general level of training.

Factors influencing the receipt of orthodontic treatment

A definite malocclusion is by no means the only factor that determines whether or not an individual receives treatment; the decision to embark upon it reflects a series of features and motives of the consumers and the providers.

Among *consumers*, the strongest motivating factor is the opportunity for an improved appearance. As noted above, the perceived acceptable or normal range of variation is fairly wide, but preoccupation with personal appearance is a common feature of contemporary affluent societies. Discrepancy between actual and perceived body image leads to discontentment and possible remedial action – a change in hair style, going on a diet, getting a tan. Being able to delegate the task of such self-improvement to a third party, such as an orthodontist, is particularly attractive. Society also places greater emphasis on maximizing attractiveness in the female than in the male, and more girls than boys receive orthodontic treatment, in spite of the fact that the prevalence of malocclusion within the sexes is the same.

In Britain and North America a large proportion of children have objectively good occlusion, but as many as 50 per cent have been found to be dissatisfied with their teeth. The explanation may lie partly in the imprecise way in which individuals perceive their own dentitions. Thus, it has been found that children's and parents' descriptions of the child's dentition from memory are generally inaccurate, and furthermore, nearly one-third of a group of children and parents were unable to identify a photograph of the child's teeth.

Referral by a dentist for orthodontic care carries with it a strong implicit message that treatment is both necessary and worthwhile. Prospective patients commonly do not even know why they have been referred. Yet in clinical practice different consumers clearly have varying levels of faith, ranging from suspicion and distrust to acceptance of virtually anything the provider suggests. Perhaps the commonest question asked of the dentist during the consultation is: 'What would you advise?' The reply is crucial. Clearly it should be intelligent, reasoned and individualized.

There are reports that 'tooth braces' are worn as a 'badge of honour' or, in settings where orthodontic treatment represents a substantial economic investment by the family, as a status symbol. For these reasons there is now, in the USA, a demand for orthodontic appliances with coloured wires.

On the *provider* side, the crucial role of the general dental practitioner in the initiation of orthodontic treatment has been demonstrated on both sides of the Atlantic. Given the unrelenting exposure of dentists, and particularly orthodontists, to 'optimal' occlusions during training, it is hardly surprising that their perceptions are generally more stringent than those of the general public. But dentists have remarkably different thresholds for treatment initiation or referral. As the 'experts' cannot agree as to what constitutes need, it is hardly surprising that individual dentists are inconsistent in their clinical decisions and expectations.

THE INCREASING INFLUENCE OF MEDICAL CARE ON DENTAL TREATMENT

(Drinnan) The old adage *primum non nocere*, which can be roughly translated 'As a first priority, do not cause harm', is ever more relevant today. Recent dramatic advances in knowledge and technique have had a profound effect on modern medical practice. Many patients who formerly would have succumbed to their diseases are now kept alive and are enjoying a comfortable and productive existence. When combined with improved social and psychological support systems, this means that there are many more elderly patients seeking dental care. Some of these people have special oral problems

that are infrequently encountered in 'younger' populations, and they are having very significant effects on the practice of dentistry. It cannot be stressed too strongly that dental practitioners should be aware of any diseases which their patients have, particularly those which may be associated with complications when dental treatment is undertaken.

The explosion in medical knowledge requires modern medical or dental practitioners to constantly update their own understanding. To foster this, many of the States of the USA now require that medical and dental licensure depends on evidence of a practitioner having participated in postgraduate continuing education. Unfortunately, however, there is much evidence to suggest that dental practitioners, at least in certain parts of the USA, have inadequate knowledge about significant contemporary medical problems. Thus, even though time in the dental curriculum is devoted to such matters as medical history-taking, soft-tissue examination and radiography, these tasks are not always undertaken routinely in practice. One investigation of dentists' knowledge about the acquired immune deficiency syndrome (AIDS) has concluded that they knew little of its oral and systemic signs and symptoms, in spite of its significance in dental practice.

How should the informed dental practitioner identify those patients with significant medical conditions? It used to be said, facetiously, that a dentist need only establish a practice up a flight of stairs in a building without a lift; any patient who arrived unaided could be considered to be in reasonable physical health! However, such a 'physical test' is of little significance nowadays. Instead, obtaining a comprehensive *medical history* is undoubtedly the most important step a dentist can take to identify the medically problematical patient. Unfortunately, many practitioners rely on anamnesic questionnaires of uncertain quality. Indeed, sometimes these are given to a patient to complete in the waiting room and are never reviewed by the practitioner directly with the patient – this can lead to serious problems.

Thus, in the Duchess County (New York) Supreme Court, $1 050 700 were awarded in 1983 against a dentist to a 22-year-old man who, it was claimed, had suffered brain damage after a dental procedure. On requesting the extraction of a painful tooth, he had been given a standard health history form. Unfortunately, he gave this to his accompanying friend to complete and no note was made of the rheumatic fever and residual heart damage from which he suffered. The dentist did not ask who had completed the form and did not review it with the patient. Consequently, the tooth was removed without any prophylactic antibiotic therapy and, three weeks after, the young man had a stroke with hemiplegia and other neurological deficits. He also developed severe heart damage and it was necessary to replace one of his heart valves with an artificial one. The pathogenesis of this disaster was believed to have been of a 'textbook' kind – bacteraemia after the extraction; bacteria lodging on the damaged heart valve; vegetations breaking off the valve; and emboli to the brain with resultant brain damage.

45

The plaintiff's attorneys argued that the dentist had been delinquent in not reviewing the health history with the patient. The case provoked much discussion among practitioners, with a Dental Society offering an *amicus curiae* brief in support of the 'generally accepted practice in which the dentist relies on the answers provided in a signed questionnaire'. The case was overturned on appeal, but it remains a most salutary reminder of the need to regard each patient as an individual, with personal questioning about their medical status set at an appropriate level.

A blank piece of paper on which is recorded a personal interview conducted by the dentist is as effective, perhaps even more effective, than any structured questionnaire. But if a questionnaire is to be used, then the dental practitioner must review each significant question with the patient to establish that he or she understands and answers reliably. After all, when a patient's mind is occupied predominantly by a dental problem, it is most unlikely that he or she will understand the significance of a question such as 'how many times a day do you urinate?'

The following questions are the minimum needed to discover most medical conditions of 'dental significance'.

— Are you currently seeing a physician and if so for what reason?

— Are you taking any medications, and if so, of what type and by whom are they being administered?

— Have you suffered from any serious medical illness, e.g., heart, chest or renal disease, etc?

— Have you ever suffered from any allergic reactions to drugs or medications, and has there ever been any untoward incident during or following dental treatment?

— Have you had any infectious disease such as hepatitis, AIDS or herpes?

— Have you ever suffered from any serious bleeding disorder?

There will, of course, be some patients with serious *systemic diseases* yet to be diagnosed. The practitioner should therefore be aware of the oral signs and symptoms of conditions such as blood dyscrasias, neoplasia and infectious diseases. In particular, oral signs are often the first indication of infection by the human immune deficiency viruses (HIV; the AIDS virus) and there are many other life-threatening systemic diseases that may first become manifest in the mouth. If the dentist is reluctant to embark on a complicated investigation, he or she should have sufficient confidence to refer the patient to a consultant or other investigator who can oversee the necessary diagnostic steps.

In view of the large number of patients taking medication, the dentist must be aware of the more commonly used drugs and be familiar with their *side-effects*, especially of those which produce oral changes or which may interact with preparations that the dentist may prescribe. A short case history illustrates how the side-effects of drugs may easily be overlooked. A patient had been wearing complete dentures successfully for several years but had noticed that the 'suction' was gradually failing and that her mouth felt a little dry. The dentist explained to her that her dentures were fine and that her 'dryness' was due to her ageing! However, upon subsequent referral to a consultant she was asked in detail about her health and volunteered that she was under the care of her physician for 'slightly high blood pressure'. She was taking: a daily diuretic – side-effect, dryness of the mouth; a tranquillizer (she was most likely worried about her high blood pressure!) – side-effect, dryness of the mouth; an antihistamine – side-effect, dryness of the mouth! Unfortunately, the first dentist had taken no drug history and had completely missed the presumptive diagnosis of 'iatrogenic dry mouth'.

Several recently introduced drugs have specific effects on the oral tissues. It is well known that phenytoin may be a growth stimulant for the gingival fibrous tissues; gingival hyperplasia may also be seen with the use of the calcium channel blocker, nifedipine (Procardia, Adalat). There are also several reports of gingival hyperplasia after the administration of the immunosuppressant, cyclosporin, which is used to avert rejection in human organ transplantation.

Having detected that a patient suffers from a significant disease, and having evaluated the health status and dental needs, the dentist should be ready to *act*. For some systemic diseases little change in routine is required. For others, relevant steps should be taken and, for serious conditions, these may be so complicated as to merit referral. Clearly, a patient receiving anticoagulant therapy who requires oral surgery will need to be managed medically; and a patient with a heart condition predisposing to an endocarditis after a 'dental bacteraemia' needs special attention. For conditions such as these, there are several published standards concerning acceptable clinical routines. While there is not agreement worldwide on the precise nature of the recommended regimens, it is generally accepted that if a practitioner follows the guidelines diligently there would be a large 'umbrella' of protection against litigation should any problem such as an endocarditis arise. It is important to note that recommendations concerning antibiotics have changed significantly over the past 10 or so years and several studies have shown that many practitioners are out of date in their use.

ORAL MUCOSAL DISEASES

(Scully) New patterns of oral mucosal disease, including new disorders, are emerging globally; their incidence is increasing, and this trend is likely to continue. Although infection with HIV and its relationship to AIDS is the

single condition likely to have the most profound impact on oral health care, other new disorders are causing changes in oral health and in the nature of care required. Immune defects, immunosuppressive and other iatrogenic diseases, and immunologically-mediated disease and infection account for most new oral mucosal entities. These will undoubtedly be of major significance in the future, placing a tremendous burden on the dental profession, not only in regard of continuing education, but also in recognizing the need for holistic patient care and an expanding dialogue with the medical profession.

The impact of HIV

(Pindborg) It took some time after 1981, when the first cases of AIDS were published, for the world to realize that it was facing a widespread epidemic of unexpected proportions. Early in that epidemic it became clear that the mouth is often the seat of pathological change in HIV infection, although again it took some time for the dental profession to appreciate the situation. This was in spite of the fact that the very first paper on AIDS mentioned that four out of five patients had oral candidiasis. Since then, it has been widely recognized that a variety of oral lesions is often present, not only in AIDS patients but also in healthy seropositives (patients having antibodies to HIV) and patients with the AIDS-related complex (ARC). Any of this multiplicity of oral lesions may act as a marker for HIV infection and some may also serve as predictors.

While oral candidiasis is one of the most common of the oral manifestations, there are extreme and inexplicable differences in its prevalence rates among different studies. Most surprising is the low reported prevalence (4 per cent) among Nairobi prostitutes with HIV; at the other extreme, it was found in 57 per cent of a group in Italy. This candidal infection may be subdivided into four types: pseudomembranous, hyperplastic, erythematous and angular cheilitis. In a Copenhagen sample, pseudomembranous candidiasis was more common in AIDS patients, whereas erythematous candidiasis was the prevalent type among asymptomatic seropositives. The simultaneous occurrence of an erythematous candidiasis in the palate and on the dorsum of the tongue, without a commissural infection, is a strong sign of seropositivity (antibody response to HIV).

The first indication of an association between HIV infection and periodontal lesions came in 1985 with a report on a high prevalence of necrotizing gingivitis (9 per cent) among homosexual men, in contrast to the normal prevalence of about 0.05 per cent. A pseudomembranous gingivitis and rapid destructive periodontitis also occur in a number of HIV patients. Prevalence figures are lacking, but clearly dentists and dental hygienists should be alert when patients present with unusual periodontal problems.

The most important viral infection developing in such patients is manifest as hairy leukoplakia, which was first described in 1984, and has now been shown to be associated with the Epstein–Barr virus (*see* p. 50). The lesions are most common bilaterally on the margins of the tongue. The predictive value of hairy leukoplakia has been demonstrated in a remarkable follow-up study from San Francisco in which it was found that the probability of AIDS developing was 48 per cent by 16 months after the leukoplakia had been diagnosed, and 83 per cent by 31 months.[34]

There are, at present, nearly 40 other oral lesions that may be seen in HIV-infected patients, and it should be emphasized in particular that oral ulcerations of unknown aetiology should raise suspicion. Clearly, the HIV epidemic has been, is and will be a great challenge to the dental profession in the years to come. The responsibility for dentists and other oral health workers concerns the ability to make an early diagnosis on the basis of oral lesions, and a duty to treat these patients. Obviously the emergence of HIV infection has led to much greater awareness of infection control, which also is of significance for preventing hepatitis B.

Immunocompromised patients

(*Scully*) Immunosuppressive agents are prescribed in the management of a wide range of diseases and they are commonly used to inhibit graft rejection and autoantibody production. Such drugs include corticosteroids, azathioprine, cyclophosphamide and cyclosporin; and this therapy predisposes to two main effects on oral mucosa and other tissues – infection and neoplasia.

Infection is the most frequent complication, especially by viruses, fungi and mycobacteria. Thus herpesvirus infection and candidiasis are common, and these organisms are found in saliva. Herpes simplex virus infections may affect most parts of the mouth as well as lead to the more typical recurrent lip lesions. Acyclovir remains the most effective therapy. Shingles (herpes varicella-zoster virus) occurs in many immunocompromised patients, especially those with Hodgkin's lymphoma, and particularly after chemotherapy and radiotherapy. In such patients, the virus may cause chickenpox even if they have had a previous attack, which normally is protective. Trigeminal zoster may cause (and be followed by) severe orofacial pain, and may lead to oral ulceration along with an ipsilateral facial rash. The immunocompromised may also develop chronic zoster infection. Immunosuppressive therapy predisposes to human papillomavirus infections, oral lesions of which are increasingly recognized.

The best known presentation of oral candidiasis is the soft, creamy plaques of thrush, typically on the soft palate or in the upper buccal sulcus. If no local cause for thrush can be found, such as medication (e.g. a corticosteroid inhaler) or xerostomia, an immune defect should be sought. In the immunocompromised, oral candidiasis may spread to the oesophagus and, in the immunosuppressed, it may disseminate and be life-threatening. During im-munosuppression, particularly in renal transplantation, patients may also acquire thrush-like oral lesions that are actually plaques of mixed bacterial origin. Dental plaque itself may come to contain atypical bacteria such as enterococci and *Capnocytophaga*, and the latter may also be disseminated systemically.

In immunocompetent people, Epstein–Barr virus infection typically pro-duces cervical lymph node enlargement, pharyngitis and fever, leading to full-blown infectious mononucleosis (glandular fever) in its most developed form, but in immunocompromised patients it may produce malignant lym-phoproliferative disorders, especially lymphomas. The virus has also been implicated in the hairy oral leukoplakia of HIV infection, and has clear associations with Burkitt's lymphoma and undifferentiated nasopharyngeal carcinoma. Immunosuppression itself produces a small but important pre-disposition to *neoplasia* – labial carcinoma, oral Kaposi's sarcoma, and lymphomas. Renal transplant patients may develop oral white lesions (kera-tosis), though these do not appear to be premalignant.

For bone marrow transplantation, which is being increasingly used in the treatment of aplastic anaemia, leukaemias, and certain immune defects, patients are usually prepared by immunosuppression with cyclophosphamide and total body irradiation. Oral symptoms are the main adverse effect of this; they include mucositis, parotitis and dry mouth, sinusitis and other infections. After the transplant, graft lymphocytes may mount an immunological attack on the recipient to produce 'graft versus host disease', characteristic features of which include lichenoid reactions of oral mucosa and/or skin, and some-times a sclerodermatous reaction with dry mouth and rampant caries. Cyclo-sporin or methotrexate may ameliorate or prevent this attack but these can also produce adverse effects – gingival hyperplasia and mouth ulcers respec-tively.

Lichen planus and lichenoid reactions

The aetiology of oral *lichen planus* (a chronic dermatosis that affects the mouth and/or skin) remains obscure,[35] but factors identifiable in a minority of patients include the 'graft versus host disease' described above, various drugs (especially the non-steroidal anti-inflammatory agents, antihypertens-ive agents, antidiabetic drugs and antimalarials), together with reactions to dental restorative materials. The pathogenesis of reactions to restorations is unclear but electrogalvanism and contact allergy[36] have been implicated. No evidence of true hypersensitivity has been found[37] and the now reported appearance of lichenoid reactions to composite restorations[38] may dampen some of the enthusiasm for the wholesale replacement of amalgams.

Immunologically-mediated and other disorders

Proven *allergic reactions* in the mouth are extremely rare but it is likely that oral manifestations of food intolerance will come to be recognized as more important than hitherto supposed.

It is now appreciated that the vesiculo-bullous (blistering) disease, *pemphigoid*, is actually a heterogeneous group of disorders. The majority of patients with oral lesions of this type may have mucous membrane pemphigoid, but this may not always be confirmed by laboratory tests and it is important to differentiate bullous pemphigoid, dermatitis herpetiformis and the linear IgA variant, as well as non-immunological disorders such as *localized oral purpura*. This bleeding disorder of unknown aetiology is fairly common, affecting predominantly middle-aged or elderly patients, and is characterized by blisters, commonly filled with blood, and often on the soft palate. Their appearance often frightens the patient but the blisters rarely occlude the airway; rather they burst within 24–48 hours to leave ulcers that heal in 7–10 days.

Infections

Increasing mobility of populations and improved air travel mean that some infectious diseases have spread, or are spreading, world-wide, thereby presenting the dentist with new challenges in diagnosis and involvement. *Oral gonorrhoea* exemplifies this situation: as with most sexually transmitted disorders, this is increasing in prevalence and will possibly continue to do so, but it is only relatively recently that it has been recognized – pharyngitis or an acute gingivitis somewhat resembling ANUG are its main features.

The use of smokeless tobacco

Smokeless tobacco is increasing in popularity in many Western countries, especially amongst the young, with whom snuff and chewing tobacco are the most common forms. There is considerable concern about the possible carcinogenicity and other adverse effects of the snuff now sold in small 'tea-bag' pouches.[39] Smokeless tobacco can also be associated with oral keratosis and possibly gingival recession; clearly, its use is to be deprecated.

4
New strategies for oral health care

Across the world a significant effort is being made to implement new and appropriate strategies for oral health care, some of which are now considered. The account moves from the generality of population-based measures to some specifics of measures devised by individual developing and developed countries.

ORAL HEALTH FOR ALL – A REALISTIC GOAL?

(Sardo Infirri) The World Health Organization has set a goal *Health for all by the year 2000*. For oral health the underlying strategy by which this goal might be achieved embraces the concept of *primary health care* – the availability of essential care *where people live and work*, together with care at the first referral level for *all* communities. It is implicit that this individual and family care should be based on practical, scientifically sound and socially acceptable methods and technology, made universally available through the full participation of the individuals in the community, and at a cost the community can afford and maintain.

(Nitisiri) It was affirmed in the declaration of Alma Ata (USSR) in 1979 that a primary health care approach is essential for achieving an acceptable level of health globally. For oral health it may be argued, simplistically, that the basic principle for success is based on self-care and self-help, which includes effective brushing of the teeth every day. Tooth brushing, of course, readily lends itself to the primary health care concept and it would, at first sight, appear to be relatively simple and feasible to implement throughout the world. However, in reality, there are many factors that inhibit this.

In industrialized countries, tooth brushing is a common practice associated with everyday living, but in developing countries it is not a standard procedure for three main reasons. First, people may not know what toothbrushes are and why they should use them. Secondly, they may know about toothbrushes but be unable to afford them; some may use other devices such as chewing sticks (*see* p. 57). This situation is quite common in countries with a low or moderate gross national product (GNP), and it should be appreciated that the traditional methods do offer some definite benefits. Thirdly, the people may be able to afford toothbrushes, knowing what they are and why they should use them, but be reluctant to do so because they may cause pain and because they feel uncomfortable about the gingival bleeding elicited by brushing. This dilemma is obviously related to the presence of periodontal disease; such people may need professional treatment to accompany their own efforts at oral health promotion.

(Sardo Infirri) How, then, can primary oral health care of any type be made realistic and relevant for those living in developing countries? Many ways of making dentistry less of a repair operation have been proposed (certain non-invasive techniques have been reviewed in Chapter 3), but these have generally been directed at improving services that people already have. For the large majority who have no access to such services, this approach is meaningless and an alternative is needed. A practical alternative is:

— The integration or re-integration of oral health into general health and primary health care, abandoning separate training and services in dentistry and so blocking further isolation of the various health professions.

— Within this integrated setting, the training of only relatively small numbers of dentists as 'oral specialists' who would work in well-designed teams to facilitate oral care; they would become leaders and planners, and would provide care at the level of final referral (mainly regionally or nationally).

— The restriction of oral care activities to:
  - health promotion through hygiene and self-care;
  - making available cheap, effective self- and family-care products, e.g. bringing fluoride toothpaste or similar agents to as many people as possible by innovative low-cost packaging and local production;
  - systematic use of non-invasive arresting and control procedures to ensure that carious lesions do not progress;
  - using extraction only as a last resort;
  - reserving oral specialities for high-quality, high-technology care, for trauma and for major pathology.

— Providing training and support to community workers and health workers, teachers, and even volunteers, so that they can provide the basic oral care measures necessary for disease prevention and control.

— Taking maximum advantage of research findings:
  - by applying new materials and products for preventing, controlling and arresting lesions;
  - by establishing community field trails to test and evaluate the cost and effectiveness of new strategies and methods;
  - by developing, through research in health services, criteria and approaches for the economic and effective use of scaling, sealants and control procedures that are often seen as only relevant in industrialized countries.

Practical steps to help effect this sort of strategy are being taken, for example by the World Health Organization, and a set of practical 'tools' is being developed for testing initially in a series of 18 projects in developing countries of Africa, South East Asia and the Eastern Mediterranean region. It comprises the following elements:

— the methodology for a community participation approach;

— a set of teaching posters, suitable for primary health workers and adults, illustrating and explaining preventive self-care aspects, self-examination and identification of the need for referral care;

— a training manual for oral health care procedures for primary health workers;

— a portable training model;

— a standard set of hand instruments;

— a clinical head rest that can be fitted to a medical examination couch or table, or indeed to any appropriate surface;

— a standard set of materials and drugs;

— a basic autoclave with cassettes for dental instruments;

— a simple storage and carrying box.

This practical package requires considerable further development, but it is certainly relevant to all developing countries and may well be of interest and use in industrialized countries as the oral care personnel become increasingly involved in community activities. Especially needed are clinical materials and drugs that prevent, arrest and control oral diseases safely *and* which are suitable for use in very differing climates and environments.

Some of the technical problems in this area are being, or will be, overcome; the crucial issue is that of creating and maintaining the political, professional and scientific will to engage in this process of change. Intensive programmes of research are also essential to develop and evaluate the cost and effectiveness of the various different activities and measures. These will ensure that the applied oral health care is culturally appropriate as well as economically feasible and maintainable within the community resources.

PRIMARY ORAL HEALTH CARE IN THAILAND

(Nitisiri) Primary health care in Thailand was started many years ago in rural areas by developing a work-force at the 'grass roots' level comprising the village health communicators and village health volunteers who promote health through organized community activities. These personnel are respon-

for carrying out packages of health measures, aimed at promoting the philosophy of self-help. Education in oral health had, for many years, been a part of one such module, but this was not comprehensive enough to solve all oral health problems. However, good progress has been made at the Intercountry Centre for Oral Health in Chiang Mai (with the collaboration and support of the World Health Organization) in carrying out research in oral health services. The project *Testing an Alternative Community Care Model in Oral Health* was established there in 1984; it is also examining a new training system for primary health workers founded on value-orientated (i.e. health-promoting) rather than technique-orientated principles.

The community care model consists of a network of oral health care services at the primary level, staffed by local residents in the sub-districts and villages – the so-called health maintenance units. This level of care comprises screening for oral conditions, oral health education, pain relief, scaling and linkage to the first referral clinic. The sub-district health workers record oral health status and prescribe drugs for pain relief. The teachers, village health volunteers and village health communicators render oral health education to the villagers. Young people in the villages are selected and trained to be 'village scalers' and scaling is done in the community on a prescription basis. Only very simple equipment, mostly made locally, is required.

A first referral clinic (health restoration centre) with five dental units has been established at the Intercountry Centre. The dentist and four auxiliaries there have been subjected to the rigorous training method known as 'performance simulation training'[40] to enable them to work logically, systematically and with a good posture. The dentist is the team leader and performs complex procedures; the auxiliaries undertake the simpler tasks, mainly fillings, extractions, endodontic treatments and simple dentures, all being arranged through an appointment system. A minibus transports villagers to this clinic. The charges for treatment are greatly subsidized; there is no service charge for primary schoolchildren but secondary schoolchildren have to pay half the standard fees.

In order to promote self-reliance in health promotion, a new study has been developed to test the feasibility of community participation through the building up of funds via the village co-operative shops. Fifteen thousand toothbrushes donated from Switzerland are to be sold, and the plan is that, in due course, the villagers who receive the scaling service will also contribute to the fund for their village. They will then be responsible for paying the salary of the scaler with the money received from shares in the co-operative shop and from the charge for scaling.

In 1986, an oral health survey that included an interim evaluation of this community care model was carried out by the Intercountry Centre in collaboration with the John J Sparkham Centre for International Public Health Education at the University of Alabama, Birmingham, USA. Gingival health was assessed by the Community Periodontal Index of Treatment Needs

(CPITN; *see* Chapter 3). In large samples of people in Samerng and Pasang, calculus made the greatest contribution to high CPITN scores. Among individuals aged 15–18 years, those who had been scaled had a higher mean number of healthy sextants than those who had not. However, there was not much difference in that mean number among adults aged 35–44 years; and the calculus scores for these people were high, whether they had been scaled or not. In spite of this, the majority of people in both villages said that they brushed their teeth two or more times a day. At least half of the subjects knew that there was a village scaler in their community, though only about a quarter had actually been scaled. About half of all respondents indicated their willingness to pay their share for the scaler's salary, but this proportion can be expected to rise markedly as the service expands, for the large majority of those who had been scaled reported satisfaction with this kind of service and were willing to make a financial contribution.

ORAL HEALTH CARE FOR THE MASSES IN INDIA

(Singh, Tiwari) In India, a vast country with a population of about 800 millions (80 per cent rural and 20 per cent urban), there has been an alarming increase in the prevalence and severity of dental caries over the last three decades. The present oral health care model is very expensive, and being orientated to treatment and rehabilitation, it cannot minimize or eliminate disease. There are approximately 10 000 dentists (1:80 000 people), 95 per cent of whom practise rehabilitative dentistry in urban areas. Forty dental schools have an intake of about 1600 students annually; 15 of these schools opened only very recently.

(Tewari, Gauba, Ashima) Rural India has a dentist : population ratio of 1:500 000 and the only viable means of providing oral health is to train those in existing health and educational infrastructure in primary preventive strategies. Indeed, the Indian Council of Medical Research, under the guidance of the Department of Dentistry at the Postgraduate Institute of Medical Education and Reasearch in Chandigarh, has formulated a plan to study the feasibility of extending primary prevention of dental caries and periodontal diseases in the community in this way. In the feasibility study, the medical doctors, various health workers and school teachers have been trained by dentists; they in turn educate the rural community and school children. Since the method has been found successful, it has formed the basis of the national plan.

To evaluate the resultant changes in knowledge, attitude and practice, various factors have been investigated at baseline and after one year. Three-quarters of the target population had been covered by oral health education programmes within that time. The proportion of adults and children using a toothbrush had increased from 30 to 41 per cent. Those using *dattan (miswak* or chewing stick) rose from 45 to 56 per cent while those using fluoride toothpaste, which in these communities is more expensive than non-fluoridated and less readily available, increased from 5 to 19 per cent.

As a result of oral health education, about one-third of the rural community and half of the children (5–16 years of age) had started to use daily 0.04 per cent fluoride mouth rinses at home, and the majority of schoolchildren were given 0.2 per cent sodium fluoride mouth rinses by their teachers every 15 days. By the end of the year, most of both the adult community and the schoolchildren had seen dental plaque in their own mouths after 'disclosing'. The Snyder lactobacillus test showed an increase from about one-third to two-thirds in the numbers of individuals graded as being in the 'zero' to 'low' caries categories, suggesting a definite change in the pattern of eating sugars.

Speeding endodontics

(Tewari, Sachdev, Kaur) The need and demand for endodontic treatment in the developing countries, and possibly in many industrialized countries, is far greater than the available facilities, manpower and resources allow. Between 1982 and 1985, in the Department of Dentistry, Chandigarh, endodontic treatment could only be provided for about a quarter of the 500–700 patients per year who sought it; and by using multi-visit endodontic sessions, the success rate was 85–90 per cent (over the first year or so). The untreated patients had teeth extracted, clearly an unsatisfactory solution. Over the last 10 years, one-visit endodontics has been promoted as the treatment of choice in very specific cases and an assessment has now begun of this procedure as a realistic public health measure.

In a prospective study over eight months, the time taken for one-visit endodontics was compared with that of multi-visit sessions, both using only the existing manpower and resources. Allocation of patients to either group was random and irrespective of clinical and radiographic diagnosis; the step-back procedure was always used for root canal preparation, followed by lateral condensation of gutta-percha. In addition to the appointment(s) for actual treatment there was, in every case, an initial visit for diagnosis and documentation, and the time taken for this was included in the total timings. For the single-visit treatments, the total time averaged 102 ± 63 minutes compared with 152 ± 45 minutes for the multi-visit procedures. The immediate success rate was 89 per cent after the single visit and 85 per cent after the multiple visits. These rates were much the same after 8–10 months. Although, the results should be viewed with some caution because of this limited follow-up time, in general terms, one-visit treatment appears efficacious for routine application, so providing considerable optimism about the possibility of endodontic therapy for all who require it, without increasing manpower or resources.

SRI LANKAN EXPERIENCES

Teaching cavity preparation to trainee school dental therapists

(Perera) Trainee school dental therapists in Sri Lanka are now being taught an updated approach to cavity preparation involving minimal tissue removal related to the extent of the caries rather than to a preconceived 'outline form'. The objective is, of course, to preserve the long-term health of the tooth and this also involves inculcating important *attitudes* – that unnecessary restorations should be avoided, applying the maxim 'when in doubt, don't cut'. The fact that many teeth, once filled, have to be repetitively restored is emphasized (*see* p. 24). It took approximately 24 hours of instruction for the students to master the minimal technique. Preliminary timings have shown that an occlusal cavity preparation took a mean of 9 minutes, while by the 'traditional' method it required a mean of 14 minutes; the equivalent times for more complex types of cavity were respectively 35 instead of 55 minutes. Treadle drills with steel burs are used.

Using the Gum Health Plan

(Warnakulasuriya, Ekanayake) The Gum Health Plan (*see* p. 14) offers a simple method for patients to detect, record and monitor their own periodontal status. It enables them to observe progress weekly and discuss the results with their dentist. The majority of patients in a Sri Lanka study had gingival bleeding at the first visit, but over half of these were free of bleeding four weeks after using the Plan. However, in its present form the method was not found acceptable to practitioners for each and every patient seen in their daily work, and so the possibility of offering it to populations directly (without the necessity for a dentist to administer or supervise it) needs to be explored.

TANZANIA – THE DEVELOPMENT OF AN ORAL HEALTH CARE SERVICE

(Luukkonen) The United Republic of Tanzania is one of the poorest developing countries in the world. Its economy is largely based on agriculture, whereas the industrial sector's share of the GNP remains around 10 per cent. Of the total population (over 20 million) about 50 per cent are children under the age of 15; the annual population growth is about 3 per cent.

(Lembariti) Tanzania inherited an inadequate health service from the past colonial system. To improve this, a pyramidal system has, more recently, been adopted. This is based on the primary health care concept, and seeks to reach the majority of the population in the rural areas. Of course, this service is still being developed, but there is already full integration of oral health into the existing general health care structure. Most of the services are implemented by the government, by government-owned companies and corporations, or by voluntary agencies, mainly religious organizations. Some 8000 village health posts form the broad base of the pyramid and four consultant hospitals the apex. The peripheral personnel are the rural medical aides and other primary health care workers at the health posts. For oral health, dental assistants, assistant dental officers and dental officers, assisted by dental auxiliaries, dental technicians and other allied health professionals, serve at the higher referral levels.

The training of the entire oral health team is conducted through the rural medical aide schools, allied health professionals' schools, teachers' colleges, two dental assistant schools, one assistant dental officer school and one dental school (described below). The educational programmes of these institutions give strong emphasis to team-work and a preventive and community orientation. Their curricula are based on the five principles of primary health care – focus on prevention, equitable distribution of services, community involvement, appropriate technology and a multisectoral approach.

The oral health care programme, embodied in Tanzania's first oral health plan, had from the beginning these objectives:

— To bring to the notice of the country's leadership and to medical professionals the importance of oral health in the development of public health. This was needed in order to obtain the necessary co-operation (in competition with other health programmes).

— To carry out national surveys that should give more reliable information regarding oral health problems.

— To promote lifestyles conducive to oral health and to change the approach of services from curative to preventive.

— To provide adequate manpower and facilities so that oral health services could be offered to the whole population.

From experience gained by the successes and failures of that first oral health plan, and from the wealth of information gathered, a new national oral health plan was launched in 1988; its main elements are now outlined.

On promoting appropriate individual and community lifestyles, the first approach was to develop individual awareness of oral diseases, and of the changes in behaviour needed to reduce self-imposed risks such as nutritional imbalance (for example, frequent sugar intakes in tea/coffee or sweets) and tobacco chewing. The existing programmes of dental health education undertaken by medical aides and teachers in primary schools are the cornerstones of this strategy, and such teaching has been extended from expectant mothers and schoolchildren into the community at large. But it is realized that broader approaches, such as arrangements to make oral hygiene implements more accessible and affordable, and to reduce the consumption of tobacco and alcohol, are also needed to improve the social and economic conditions that influence choice in lifestyle. Legislative and regulatory controls may be required to limit the sale of certain items to young people. There is, of course, considerable interdependence upon measures taken in other major sectors such as economic, water supply and food.

From the start of the first plan, the 12-year-old schoolchildren had been a priority group, while all primary and secondary schoolchildren, and expectant mothers, had been targeted as far as possible. It was now felt that those with scores for decayed, missing and filled teeth of two standard deviations higher than the national average should be given special priority for preventive and curative services. The identification of this group is therefore essential to the provision of selective treatment, and necessitates regular inspections. It is hoped to provide curative interventions, such as the filling of occlusal cavities where necessary, as part of a package designed to help all 12-year-olds maintain their oral health.

A basic objective is to train a variety of health workers in oral health care. In particular, continuing efforts are being made to ensure that all medical aides include oral health education in their regular activities, and to this end all rural dispensaries and other health facilities where these aides work are being equipped with appropriate audiovisual equipment. Although the rural medical aides are now being taught to provide basic emergency oral health care, it should be pointed out that the majority are still not doing so. The cause is partly lack of suitable equipment, and partly lack of motivation. As a consequence, the higher levels of staff, e.g. district and regional dental officers, are undertaking a disproportionate amount of minor emergency treatment.

The improvement of existing services through provision of better equipment and materials is inevitably a rather sensitive issue because it involves financial strategy. To address this problem, certain guidelines have been laid down, including:

— The use of appropriate technology: that is, technology designed for conditions found in a developing country. Thus, for example, simplified dental units are being evaluated, dental school staff are researching materials appropriate for the climate and, through the support of the Finnish International Development Agency (FINNIDA), experiments have been conducted on ultra-conservative methods of cavity preparation using only hand instruments. *Appropriate technology does not mean second-hand technology.*

— Use of only a limited range of equipment brands to reduce the problems of spares and supplies.

— Preparation of standardized lists of materials to ensure that those imported are uniform and costs thereby contained.

Creating local expertise in oral health

In the 1970s, Tanzania decided to take as much responsibility as possible for creating her own local expertise in oral health. *(Luukkonen)* Dental caries seemed to be on the increase especially among urban and young groups; periodontal diseases, oral manifestations of systemic diseases, oral cancer of various types, and oro-facial trauma from an increasing number of traffic accidents were all reported with alarming frequency. The dental manpower at that time comprised about 16 dentists and 48 dental assistants. As the estimated population was slightly over 15 million, each dentist had, on average, to look after the oral health of 1 million people. The World Health Organization recommendation was 1:20 000.

The few Tanzanian dentists in the country had been trained abroad, mostly in Western countries. Experience had shown, as it had in other countries, that direct transfer of trained manpower or the use of training programmes from the developed world are not necessarily successful as these had not been geared to the oral health needs, the community requirements or the economic reality of a poor country. Although the graduates were excellent dentists in their own right, their commitment to the promotion of oral health in Tanzania left a good deal to be desired. The output of Tanzanian dentists from foreign universities had also for years been neither sufficient nor consistent. Many of those who had graduated never returned to stay permanently in the country. For these reasons, the government established the dental school at the University of Dar es Salaam in 1979,

The degree course

(Lembariti) The Doctor of Dental Surgery degree was initiated to provide oral health personnel qualified to plan independently and execute oral health programmes, and undertake research. The needs of the society were the primary determinants of the curriculum; thus the training objectives were to incorporate oral health into general health. Bearing in mind that rapid societal changes might occur, the curriculum was designed to be dynamic and based on principles rather than merely emphasizing specific techniques. The underlying philosophy was that dental problems should be tackled through a preventive and community-orientated approach. Dental science and oral public health underpin the course, and preventive and community dentistry

account for about a quarter of the total teaching load. Every effort is made to ensure that the undergraduate does not become orientated simply towards the repair of disease. Indeed, the course promotes an understanding of the importance of organizing a comprehensive, community oral health service. It emphasizes positive promotion of oral health through education, motivating dental personnel to feel responsible for the community rather than to wait for the patient to come for treatment. Emphasis is laid on professional leadership of oral health teams in the districts, and the need for continuous training and supervision is stressed. Teachers also try to inculcate an understanding of the country's economic constraints.

The Morogoro Rotation

The facilities of the dental school are complemented by the Morogoro Rotation in primary health care, about 200 km west of Dar es Salaam. This is an urban and rural field centre for developing, monitoring and evaluating preventive and community dental activities. It involves all the members of the dental team and also serves as a base for dental research. The theoretical knowledge gained at the dental school is used here to provide oral health education to villagers, primary school pupils, secondary school students, mothers attending maternal and child health clinics, industrial workers, etc. The activities of one rotation of dental personnel are repeated in the next, and an attempt is made to measure the effects of the rotations on oral health education, through the completion of a questionnaire and an assessment of the population's oral health status. Whenever dental treatment is indicated in the population visited, it is provided at the site.

Independence and self-reliance

(*Luukkonen*) To compensate for the shortage of national academic staff, the university authorities in Dar es Salaam initially sought outside co-operation with certain European countries including Finland. Inter-university co-operation began in 1979 with teaching staff from the University of Kuopio being recruited to participate as teachers in Tanzania. The second phase of co-operation was aimed at developing the dental school towards independence in its training and research functions. The emphasis moved to postgraduate teaching, while all undergraduate teaching was gradually taken over by the national staff. Postgraduate training programmes were launched and junior academic staff started their postgraduate studies at the University of Dar es Salaam. Training was aimed at career development to prepare these staff to take full responsibility for the dental school in senior positions, so a research and scientific orientation was stressed throughout the postgraduate courses. A social research project (the Ilala Oral Health Survey) formed an integral part of the training. The third phase of co-operation, starting in 1989, will eventually complete the project cycle in 1991. This will concentrate on the training of trainers and research staff, so that the dental school will eventually have a full complement of national, highly qualified, experts. Tanzania will have reached independence and self-reliance in oral health training, research and service.

(Lembariti) It is worth noting that the dental school has the capacity to train 25 graduates per year but only 10 are needed annually for Tanzania alone. As there is a shortage of qualified manpower in oral public health in this part of Africa, the doors have been opened to admit an increasing number of students from neighbouring countries. The disease patterns, needs and common interests are more or less the same throughout the region, and the philosophy and curriculum of the school have been internationally acknowledged. There is thus considerable optimism for the future.

THE ROLE OF THE DENTAL THERAPIST IN PAPUA NEW GUINEA

(Howden) A high prevalence of dental disease, a shortage of dentists and/or money has led Governments, even in developed countries, to provide dental care by means of dental therapists and similar paradental operatives. In a 2-year course, therapists are trained in Papua New Guinea to carry out primary preventive care and various treatments for both children and adults, comprising most of the dental treatment carried out in the country. They are taught to give both infiltration and block local anaesthesia, to extract teeth and roots with forceps, and to give oral hygiene instruction and dental education both to individuals and groups, including school teachers. They are also taught to diagnose common oral diseases and to recognize and refer the abnormal. They provide scaling, but not root planing; and routine conservation, but not endodontics.

After graduation, the therapists are assigned to a regional dental clinic to work under the supervision of the regional dental officer. While at the clinics, they are also very much involved in joint patrols with the dental and medical officers to the more remote villages where mobile joint clinics are set up and dental examinations and treatment are provided.

The importance of the dental officers in the provision of the services provided by the therapists cannot be over-emphasized. They organize the clinics in terms of patients, equipment and ordering of materials, and they supervise the standard of work carried out. However, on occasions when no dental officer has been present for some reason, it has often been observed that very little work is done in the clinics. Also, mobile joint patrols cannot be organized, and visits to local schools and communities rarely take place.

Indeed, the provision of dental care in the absence of a well-motivated, energetic and determined dental officer is very limited. Clearly, lack of motivation on the part of the therapists is an important issue, and the matter is made worse by the heat and humidity.

Nevertheless, the advantages of providing dental care by dental therapists are enormous, especially in developing countries where there is a grave shortage of people with secondary education. The 2-year therapy course costs the government about a quarter of the outlay involved in training a dentist, and the salaries are less than half. If the obvious problems can be addressed and overcome, then the use of dental therapists in the provision of dental manpower is to be highly recommended, especially in developing countries.

LEARNING FROM ORAL HEALTH CARE IN THE USSR

(*Kuzmina*) Oral health care in the USSR is an integral part of the state public health system, provided at national, regional and community levels. Services are free of charge and available to all at dental clinics and at dental units affiliated to day-care centres, schools and workplaces.

As part of continuing education, stomatologists are required to take refresher courses, and there is an increasing number of qualified oral health specialists providing improved diagnosis and treatment, with updated equipment. Despite these improvements, however, there is a growing incidence of oral diseases. Epidemiological studies, which since 1983 have conformed to World Health Organization standards, show that the prevalence and severity of caries in 12-year-old children vary widely across the country. For example, the mean decayed, missing and filled index is low in Armenia, moderate in Moscow, and very high in Latvia. Caries prevalence appears to be increasing in northern parts of the country and in Eastern Siberia, while in cities like Moscow and Leningrad it is declining. On the whole, the last 10 years have witnessed some stabilization in caries incidence with a slight increase in rural areas. A CPITN study (*see* p. 13) of gingival bleeding and calculus in 15-year-old children has shown that periodontal disease in this age group is generally of high severity everywhere.

Implementation of prevention

A 5-year oral health programme has recently been developed and implemented in five cities (Moscow, Leningrad, Kiev, Riga, Odessa). Target groups include pregnant women, pre-school and school-age children, teenagers and adults, the aim being to study the effectiveness of preventive measures – dental education, oral hygiene instruction and various combinations of remineralization agents.

The level of motivation has varied: pregnant women and pre-school children were eager to participate, but the other groups seemed reluctant. The effectiveness of the measures was also variable. The average caries level for children and teenagers has dropped by 30–40 per cent, while the incidence of early, 'white spot' lesions in pregnant women has decreased to 60–80 per cent of its former level. The rest of the group of adults has improved periodontal status, but practically no changes in caries severity. As a result of this experience, the Ministry of Public Health has endorsed a number of similar programmes at the national level. But their implementation is a long and complex process, and it should be acknowledged that it does not succeed everywhere. However, the general trend gives rise to optimism, and more and more people are becoming involved.

The involvement of non-dental personnel in these primary prevention programmes has been central to their establishment. Thus, the programmes at all levels have been developed and administered under the supervision of the chief paediatrician, and the health institutions concerned are:

- out-patient departments for children;

- women's consultation centres;

- dental clinics;

- sanitary-epidemiological stations;

- health education centres;

- school and pre-school institutions.

Preventive measures are carried out by:

- paediatricians;

- obstetricians;

- gynaecologists;

- nurses;

- pre-school and school teachers;

- social workers and parents.

Within this structure the stomatologists' responsibilities are:

- to provide instruction for medical and non-medical personnel;

- to monitor preventive measures;

- to manage the secondary prevention of early caries and periodontal diseases through regular care.

The Kaunas programme

Oral health projects may be developed independently, or they may be incorporated into a wider health programme, as exemplified by the Kaunas Comprehensive Health Programme for the prevention of non-infectious diseases, introduced in 1982. After all, methods required for the prevention of common dental diseases are, in essence, similar to those used for the prevention of non-infectious diseases.

A number of oral health risk factors are taken into account within the structure of the Kaunas programme, such as excessive sugar consumption and harmful oral habits. The top priority for both the oral and general health service is to eliminate these factors. The measurable goals for oral health for the year 2000 are:

— A decrease in the decayed, missing and filled index to 3.0 for 80 per cent of 12-year-old children in the town (the index average was 4.9 in 1982).

— A reduction in the severity of periodontal diseases among 15-year-old children to a mean of not more than 2 sextants affected (in 1982 the mean was 4.5 sextants).

The preventive activities fostered are promotion of a healthy way of life, including effective oral hygiene; regulation of sugar intake; and the use of fluorides (fluoride toothpaste and mouthwash, etc.) and the remineralizing solution, 'Remodent'.

The chief stomatologists at the dental clinics supervise and control the various activities and see that primary preventive oral care activities are provided on time and at the proper level. The teachers in day-care centres provide oral hygiene instruction courses with daily participation over 2–3 weeks, followed by a repeat instruction in 2–3 months if necessary. Teachers themselves receive instruction in oral hygiene techniques from a supervising stomatologist. For schoolchildren oral hygiene instruction is carried out by teachers as part of the normal education programme; parents may also be involved. In addition, instruction and fluoride treatments are provided by school dentists and nurses at the various oral care units. Health education for the entire population is also a responsibility of the media: radio, television and newspapers carry regular features providing information on preventive action for oral health.

Over the first six years of the project there has been a drop of 30–40 per cent in the severity of dental caries and periodontal diseases among children. This first experience of mass dental prevention in the USSR augments that gained in a number of other countries in suggesting that a top priority for raising the quality of oral health care in the community is to ensure the wide application of preventive programmes.

ORAL HEALTH IN THE WORKPLACE AND COMMUNITY

(Bornstein, Zimmerman, Martinsson) A project in which oral health care is offered to employees at their place of work is in progress at three companies in Stockholm. The Swedish dental services are among the most comprehensive in the world but, although nearly all children see a dentist regularly, adults have not been reached in a systematic way. In fact, approximately one-third of the 20–60 year age group are not regular dental attenders yet caries and periodontal diseases affect a large number of them. Bringing oral health care to the workplace, via a mobile clinic that can be set up in half an hour in any available area, e.g. a conference room, has had a remarkable effect in changing this situation. During the first year, 95 per cent of all employees participated in an oral health programme, which included 6-monthly screening, preventive and emergency treatment.

So far the results have been very encouraging. For instance, a 70 per cent reduction in the prevalence of periodontal pockets deeper than 5 mm was seen after 24 months. The programme is also assisting the anti-smoking campaign, giving dietary information, screening for serious oral mucosal diseases, identifying environmental factors that affect oral health, and reaching patients who are afraid of dentistry. The simple technology involved could easily be adapted for use in developing countries.

(Zimmerman, Bornstein, Martinsson) Another Swedish initiative has been the development of outreach preventive programmes for refugee populations within the community. Twelve per cent of the Swedish population are immigrants. These include refugees from Chile, a random sample of whom were found to require a median of 6.6 hours of dental treatment. One-visit and two-visit preventive programmes were instituted and, after six months, there were substantial improvements in periodontal health, the largest effect being obtained after the first visit.

CONCLUSIONS

The daily round of routine dental practice can bring with it a distancing from other health care professionals at the community level, as well as the inevitable degree of insularity at the level of the whole profession imposed by national boundaries. The conclusion that much can be learned from approaches to oral health care in different countries is not intended to be didactic. Such learning is a two-way process, and the key-word is 'appropriateness'. It may be that the concept of primary health care as it applies to dentistry is not yet readily understood in many parts of the world. Certainly, it is easy to see how certain aspects of dental practice militate against community involvement at the primary level. The effects this will have on the future organization of oral health care is part of the theme of the next chapter.

5
Planning for the future

PREDICTIONS

(Barmes) In turning attention to the future, it is worthwhile noting at the outset that the oral health sector of medicine has not done badly in terms of prevention and care, whatever criticisms may have been advanced in earlier chapters. However, there is still great need for change to make such care appropriate and, in spite of many warnings, it seems clear that the rate of change is far too slow. The following predictions are firmly rooted in fact and provide some measure of the scene that will unfold before today's dental tyro.

If we take the year 2025 as a benchmark, the first-year dental student of 1990 will only be 55 years old, living in populations with an average life expectancy that might easily have reached 90 years in the most developed countries. It is reasonable to surmise that, in such countries, pulp-involving caries will be almost unknown in persons less than 25 years of age; it will be rare even up to 40 years. Most procedures related to caries in those age groups will have become *home-based*: the home application of fluorides and of preventive materials, such as sealants and remineralizing agents, but in simpler forms than those of today and more effective. Oral health personnel may have some duties in non-invasive care using such materials, together with the invasive restoration of carious teeth, though not much more often than for treatment of periapical granulomas today.

Also, in people up to the age of 40 years, it is difficult to believe that periodontal care will need to be any more frequent than that of caries. Either hygiene will be effective enough to prevent most bleeding and calculus, or there will be a topical preparation that will prevent calculus formation. It seems likely that most destructive forms of periodontal disease will be preventable, leaving only the residual forms for special, perhaps as yet unknown, types of care.

Extractions because of disease will be even more rare, although teeth will, of course, still have to be removed on account of lack of space in the dental arches. Orthodontic treatment will, surely, have been rationalized, but it is not possible to predict whether it will be more or less frequently applied than it is today. Apart from a few complete dentures, prosthetic care will mainly be of the fixed variety, and implants may be in widespread use. But, having risen to a peak in the first quarter of the 21st century, prosthetic treatment should be about to wane in quantity by 2025.

It is to be hoped that the 'oral physician' will have become a reality by that time. This designation (developed further on p. 77) is central to the necessary evolution from reparative, treatment-based dentistry to comprehensive, prevention-orientated oral health care. The oral physician will be the professional caring for the less common but more serious forms of oral disease and concentrating on the promotion of healthy lifestyles, integrated with action in other areas of health. It seems likely that this highly trained person will delegate such simple operative procedures as are then required to some kind of 'auxiliary' personnel. Thus, as stated elsewhere:[41]

although demographic and lifestyle changes in the populations may buffer the effect for two or three decades, the ultimate situation will be a reduced overall need for oral health care, plus a polarizing of that need towards self-care and minimal simple intervention, on the one hand, and high-technology care, on the other. An estimate of the enormity of this situation can be given in terms of full-time equivalents for personnel categories directly treating the public in highly industrialized countries. This estimate suggests that some time in the next 40 years the present total of about 650 000 such personnel will have to be reduced to about 150 000, provided there is no extension of their duties into other areas and that they are working at full capacity.

The changes that have taken place in recent years in treatment methods, materials and equipment have to be seen within the context of a range of some 40 years between the youngest and the oldest cohorts of dentists. This means that unless continuing education and relicensing are seen as essential and are carefully planned, the whole care package can never be, and never has been, highly relevant in a changing world. For there to be relevance in oral health and care by 2025, the need for systematic and co-ordinated change is clear. Thoughts will need to be focused upon:

— how to make these major changes;

— how to synchronize them in training institutions and service settings;

— how to integrate oral care activities within the whole health team;

— how to provide for complete community coverage in these new circumstances.

It is not irrational, indeed it is encouraging to believe that, through partnership of the World Health Organization with the Fédération Dentaire Internationale and the mechanism of the International Development Programme, there is the potential to involve the whole profession in these changes. However, the leadership will have to be imaginative and strong if the required cohesion is to replace the fragmentation of effort with which the profession has recently lived.

CHANGE TOWARDS PREVENTION IN THE UK

(Downer) When the National Health Service (NHS) came into being in 1948, a comprehensive dental service was included from the outset as part of

the overall provision of medical services. Now, 40 years on, the changing concepts and philosophies of dental care are necessarily being translated into new policy objectives and strategies. The substantial improvements in dental health that have taken place in the UK, together with the increasing orientation of both the profession and the public towards prevention, encouraged the Department of Health and Social Security in 1980 to set up the Dental Strategy Review Group from within the profession to examine the development of policy, and in particular a preventive strategy.[42] The Group adopted the aim of 'providing the opportunity for everyone to retain a healthy functional dentition for life, by preventing what is preventable and by containing the remaining disease (or deformity) by the efficient use and distribution of treatment resources'. This accords well with modern concepts of the purpose of a publicly financed dental care system.

Preventive dentistry, as illustrated in Chapter 4, falls largely within the purview of primary dental care. In order to understand and put into context recent policy developments aimed at promoting prevention in the future, it is helpful to have some knowledge of the essential features of the two primary dental care services, the General Dental Service and the Community Dental Service.

Over 80 per cent of the UK dental workforce is engaged in the General Dental Service, which is financed through central taxation (70 per cent in 1988), supplemented by direct charges (30 per cent) raised from patients who are not subject to exemption or remission. This demand-based service for all age groups is provided by general practitioners who are independent contractors to the NHS and who are generally paid on a fee-for-item-of-service system of remuneration, though working in their own privately owned practices. By contract, a dentist's obligation to a patient is discharged once the patient has been rendered dentally fit on completion of a discrete course of treatment (some changes in this arrangement are under discussion).

The complementary Community Dental Service is salaried and responds to the needs of priority groups including babies and children, and expectant and nursing mothers. In addition, there is an increasing commitment to all groups who experience difficulty in obtaining treatment elsewhere, including handicapped adults and the aged in institutions. As well as offering treatment in public clinics and health centres, the Community Dental Service organizes educational and therapeutic preventive programmes for groups of children at risk, and undertakes mass screening of children in schools. The present thrust of government policy is that the treatment of children should in future be undertaken in most parts of the country by general dental practitioners working in the General Dental Service but with the Community Dental Service concentrating its efforts on screening and providing treatment and group preventive programmes in areas with poor dental health.

After comprehensive review, the Government published a proposal in November 1987[43] for improving all aspects of primary health care. Entitled

Promoting Better Health, this document set out, among other things, the next stages for implementing prevention in the UK dental services, the general objectives being to:

— make the services more responsive to the needs of the consumer;

— raise standards of care;

— promote health and prevent illness;

— improve value for money.

In promoting the move from a restorative to a preventive approach, two themes are especially relevant: changing the way in which general dental practitioners are paid; and instilling a fully up-to-date treatment philosophy among them.

It is widely recognized that the method by which dentists are rewarded for their services is a powerful determinant of the content of the care they provide (*see* p. 9). In relation to this, an experimental capitation system of remuneration has been initiated for the care of children and this represents one of the most significant events affecting the General Dental Service since its inception. Under capitation, the dentist is paid a fixed annual fee for maintaining each of his or her child patients in a state of dental health. The main advantages are that capitation gives the dentist more clinical freedom, promotes prevention and innovation, and discourages over-treatment. It should also promote greater continuity of care, encouraging a long-term view of the patient's dental health. In so doing, it is also likely to increase both consumer and professional satisfaction, while its relative administrative simplicity may bring about some cost savings.

After a pilot feasibility study covering some 19 000 children and involving 50 dentists,[44] a 3-year controlled experiment was started in the autumn of 1986 in four matched pairs of contrasting areas of the country. With the agreement of a majority of local dentists, each matched pair of areas was randomized to form a capitation group of practices and a control group continuing on fee-for-item-of-service. Over 100 000 children are involved, and the care is being evaluated in cost-benefit terms. If the experiment is successful, the Government intends to give all children the opportunity of being treated on a capitation fee basis. The long-term implications for dental care in the UK could be profound.

Formal and widespread recognition that premature or inappropriate surgical intervention in the treatment of dental disease is indeed a problem (*see* Chapter 3) should, in itself, help promote the desired evolution from a restorative to a preventive philosophy. This recognition came in 1984 when the Minister for Health set up a Committee of Enquiry into Unnecessary Dental Treatment in response to media, consumer, professional and parliamentary concern. The committee concluded, among other things, that there was a large amount of unnecessary treatment being carried out which was attributable to an out-of-date treatment philosophy.[45] Among the many detailed recommendations in the report was an item concerning the need for greater co-operation between appropriate bodies in establishing standards of good clinical practice to be applied throughout the profession. The need to encourage dentists to undergo regular updating courses also rang through strongly, together with the need to consider ways in which the teaching of diagnostic skills might be improved in the dental schools. Action on these educational recommendations has included greatly increased financial provision for continuing education, and the Government is considering ways of rewarding dentists who undertake postgraduate training to update their knowledge and skills. Among other specific initiatives, a programme of distance learning via videos delivered free to all dental practices was launched in 1988.

Against a steadily improving environmental background, many other changes are taking place which are either directly or indirectly beneficial. These include the provision of specific preventive items in the General Dental Service fee scale, and action (closure of dental schools) to slow down the growth of dental manpower. At the same time, the public, the ultimate beneficiaries, are more dentally aware than ever before and there is an important change of attitude toward the value of preserving a natural dentition.

ORAL HEALTH AND THE AWARE CONSUMER

(Sheiham) Certain consumer trends are having a significant impact on oral health and will continue to do so in the future. For example, there is far greater emphasis on self-care and healthier lifestyles; fitness, body shape, heart disease, blood pressure and cancer have become dominant health concerns for many individuals. This has led to dietary changes, including reduced consumption of sugars and a quest for natural foods free of additives.[46] The impact on future patterns of dental caries of a reduction by half in the level of sugars' consumption, the common objective of most food and health policies, would be considerable. Aware consumers are smoking and drinking less, and more people are alert to measures that may curtail unproductive stress. Health promotion is generally perceived as making healthier choices the easier choices. Self-examination and self-care are combined, for some, with a growing sceptism about the intrusive and excessively technological aspects of Western medicine and dentistry.

(Midda) If the dental profession is to acknowledge more fully the consumers of its services, it also has a duty to be realistic in the advice it gives them. Traditional guidelines like: 'Brush after every meal', 'Don't eat sweets' and 'Visit the dentist every six months to prevent decay' may be inadequate. Food does not *cause* caries – it only has a cariogenic potential, which will be

modified by numerous other factors in the mouth. (Whether cariogenic potential is high or low is, of course, of central importance). Thus, in a clean mouth sugar is unlikely to be as 'harmful' as in a dirty mouth. Further, the over-simplistic view that sucrose is the arch villain in the promotion of caries must be questioned for, potentially, all the simple sugars are cariogenic in the mixed bacterial flora of human plaque. Thus the substitution of sucrose by any of the other sugars, either from natural or manufactured products, is no way to prevent the disease. It has to be accepted that people will seek sweetness for a variety of reasons, and any method of preventive advice that curtails pleasure is unlikely to be followed. The consumer needs *full* information before being able to make an educated dietary choice in relation to dental health. While a well-balanced diet can be achieved in three meals a day, most people in the UK and elsewhere elect to eat on at least two other occasions, thus resulting in five or more daily challenges to the teeth. A recent survey showed that 30 per cent of the energy requirement of children in the UK was obtained from snacking; clearly any preventive dental advice should bear this in mind.

In the personal view of this contributor, as far as any acceptable advice may be summarized at this stage, it would be to urge:

— the removal of plaque from each surface of each tooth at least once a day;

— fortification with fluoride (daily for all people of all ages);

— avoidance of frequent snacking;

— visit the dentist for a health check.

Increasingly consumers will come to realize that they are responsible for their own oral health and that the dentist is their guide and counsellor to help them achieve this.

One may suppose that even relatively minor innovations, *(Gazi, Moran)* such as the finding of antiplaque features in *Acacia arabica* chewing gum, a 'natural' product, may appeal to many of today's consumers. Acacia gum consists primarily of arabica, which is a complex mixture of calcium, magnesium and potassium salts of arabic acid. It has been used for thousands of years as an astringent, to cover inflamed and burned surfaces, and for checking epistaxis; now its possible future use in toothpaste and mouthrinse formulae is being actively investigated.

CHANGES IN DENTAL PRACTICE

(Sheiham) From all that has been said above, it is obvious that the recent and welcome dramatic improvements in oral health in most industrialized countries will markedly alter future patterns of dental practice, although

perhaps the profound implications of these changes have received insufficient attention. There have already been reactive rather than pro-active changes in the pattern of dental practice. The most significant of these are:

— fewer extractions and fewer dentures;

— less routine operative dentistry (conservation);

— more crowns, bridges and endodontics; more periodontal treatment; more orthodontics.

Together, these have led to a greater emphasis on diagnosis and (at least in the UK) to a decrease in the amount and cost of work done per course of treatment. The most dramatic changes concern schoolchildren, and these are particularly marked in countries with organized school dental care provided by salaried staff. In the School Dental Service in New Zealand, for example, there has recently been a reduction of 47 per cent over three years in the annual number of restorations in permanent teeth.

In the immediate future, then, dentistry faces a more critical public – one with an increased desire for dental health. Greater awareness and knowledge about health, together with more understanding of the potential hazards of cross-infection, will lead to demands for better and more time-consuming dentist–patient interaction. These factors are, in turn, likely to decrease the demand for itemized dental treatment.

Where the incidence of dental caries and the need for restorative care continue to decline, as is likely in the UK, the proportion of teeth that are sound will rise progressively in the population as successive cohorts of relatively caries-free children become adults. At the same time, it has been estimated that in England and Wales the numbers of teeth present and therefore at risk of disease in adults will increase from 700 million in 1978 to 1000–1200 million in the year 2018. There may therefore be a small increase, over the next 40 years or so, in the need for complex restorative procedures and endodontics, especially among older people, but this increase is unlikely to match the decrease in the need for basic restorations. What caries there is, is likely to continue to be skewed in incidence by socio-economic factors (*see* p. 23).

In industrialized countries, use of improved oral diagnostic methods should soon become widespread; in particular, there are likely to be significant improvements in computer-aided dental radiographic techniques and in alternatives to ionizing radiation. The greater application of innovative adhesive restorative systems (*see* also Chapter 3), involving less loss of sound tooth substance, may reasonably be expected to result in restorations with considerably increased durability. These, together with less secondary caries, are further likely to reduce the need for complex restorations later in life. It follows that the need for full or partial dentures should decline rapidly.

The intervals between recalls for re-examination for much of the population will increase as understanding about the rates of progression and the prevention of caries and periodontal diseases becomes common knowledge and as the prevalence of these diseases declines further. Some countries already have 12- or 18-month recall intervals as standard. Suitable intervals between examinations for children will focus on at-risk groups rather than rely on a rigid recall formula for all. (*Lester*) In the context of Australian experience, the following is a reasonable summary of recommended recall intervals.

— Major examinations should be made at the ages of 2, 6 and 12 years.

— In addition, *minor* recall examinations should be made at 12-month intervals for patients in non-fluoridated areas and at 18-month intervals (with certain occlusal assessments at 8 and 10 years) for patients in fluoridated areas, though at 6-month intervals where the patient has persistently poor oral health.

This latter recommendation includes children suffering from feeding bottle or 'nursing' caries, concern about which has prompted elsewhere the suggestion for routine dental examinations at 1 year of age.[47] (*MacIntyre*) Nursing caries can be a serious problem: a survey at Ad-Dammam, Kingdom of Saudi Arabia, included assessment of caries prevalence in the deciduous upper incisors at 3–5 years of age, a manifestation which is known to be associated with 'on demand' breast or bottle feeding 24 hours a day up to about 3 years of age. One-third of the children had evidence of nursing caries, often rampant.

(*Sheiham*) On the other hand, when caries rates are low, there should be a selective reduction in certain preventive measures, such as professionally applied fluoride and fluoride rinses, as these will be seen not to be cost-effective. Conversely, an increase (from existing low levels) in fissure sealing can be predicted; this will come to be a potent preventive and therapeutic measure. An appreciation that periodontal disease need only be a minor problem for the majority of people will become disseminated as improvements in general and oral cleanliness, and reductions in tobacco smoking, come to exert their full effects on periodontal health.

Supply and demand

The above factors are likely to lead to a very real discrepancy between the numbers, types and functions, distribution and quality of oral health workers on the one hand, and on the requirements for their services on the other. In most developed countries, the organized dental profession is, perhaps understandably, making efforts to increase the utilization of dental services. And stimulation of demand can be expected to have some of the desired beneficial effect, provided that dentists can re-orientate their practices and attitudes to the wants of the public. Unless they do so, growing public sceptism about the product being marketed, lower perceived needs and rising costs are likely to lead to a decline in demand, and to longer intervals between recalls, but for the wrong reasons.

The gap between the need for and supply of professional dental services has closed rapidly in some industrialized countries; in others there is already a significant oversupply of dentists. Where this occurs, there may be a strong temptation for practitioners to carry out unnecessary dental treatment when their appointment books are not full.[45] *(Tala)* The risk of unnecessary treatment must therefore be taken into *serious* consideration during the next few decades, especially when it is realized that many of today's young dentists still feel most comfortable undertaking restorative care. *(Sheiham)* However, any tendency to over-treat should be countered, at least in part, by increased consumer awareness, rising treatment costs and closer monitoring of treatment by third-party payment organizations.

Changes in education and personnel

(Johnson) Scientific developments in understanding oral diseases lend weight to the developing argument for a smaller dental profession, the members of which will become oral physicians (*see* p. 99) working as leaders of teams of auxiliaries. They will have to be educated more profoundly than before. A thorough knowledge of the basic sciences, and of pathology, medicine and pharmacology, will be required in order to put into effect and interpret diagnostic and prognostic tests, especially those involved in screening for risk of disease, which are likely to become major activities of general practice. Much of specialization should move to a postgraduate period. This confirms the need for vocational and continuing education, which appears now to be well recognized. The case for such evolutionary development was made as long as two decades ago[48] and the arguments in favour of it are now overwhelming.

More specialist knowledge will be required so that those with advanced disease or the complications of past failures in treatment can be adequately and skilfully dealt with. Certainly, there is likely to be a growing need for the oral management of patients with medical complications (*see* Chapter 4). The types and depths of specialization within dentistry may thereby grow, but there may not be a need for a marked growth in the actual numbers of specialists in the industrialized countries.

Changes in formal dental education must originate in the degree course (as illustrated by the Tanzanian experience, p. 62). Other current tentative attempts at innovation may be cited. For example, *(Lester)* the University of Sydney dental faculty is examining the feasibility of a common first-tier degree in biological sciences with the medical faculty prior to clinical training.

This approach is the direct opposite of the thrust for clinical integration with the basic sciences that has been the object of action for the last 10 years or so. The hope is that it will result in a more scientifically based and mature student for the subsequent clinical experience, as flexibility and sensitivity may well be the watchwords for the future. Pleas have already been made[49] for combining, in a geographical and administrative sense, the increasingly fragmented remnants of dental education and training for all members of the dental team. This remains a formidable political challenge.

(Sheiham) One obvious conclusion, already outlined above, must be that as well as a change in professional attitudes and education there is a need for a phased reduction in the production of dentists, together with incentives for early retirement and redeployment. For example, the British Dental Association Manpower Subcommittee has considered that it may be necessary to plan for a substantial future shrinkage (*see* p. 70) in the stock of dentists. Such reduction implies more people per dentist. Generally, dentist-to-population ratios of 1:4000 are envisaged if no auxiliaries are used, or 1:12 000 with two operating auxiliaries, assuming that 30 minutes of care will be provided per person per year. There will be a decrease in the frequency of need for what may be called medium-tech dental treatment (e.g. conventional restorations) and an increase in both low-tech (e.g. counselling) and high-tech (e.g. fixed prostheses) applications and skills. The use of auxiliaries for low-tech tasks may well become essential in order to contain costs, in which case their numbers are bound to increase.

Having said this, it should certainly also be acknowledged that most estimates of dental need are likely to be incorrect, for they are based on questionable criteria for disease.[50] Yet any predictions concerning future practice must largely be based on perceptions of future need, because existing estimates of demand are themselves of especially doubtful validity.

(Tala) The tradition of having dentists as the main component of the dental workforce should therefore be changed into an 'onion-shaped' profile, on the top of which are oral physicians, in the middle oral hygienists (and technicians), and at the bottom, oral health assistants. The middle level workforce should bear the main responsibility for health promotion and prevention. The number of oral health assistants could be one-and-a-half to two times as large as that of oral physicians.

Planning is essential to any change in the patterns of dental practice. It will provide a stimulating challenge for those who are adequately prepared to be accommodated into the future oral health care system, integrated as it should be into primary health care. There is currently some complacency in various quarters about the need to change the pattern of dental practice and dental education, reinforced by discussions of unmet need and the stimulation of demand, but this reaction is surely short-sighted? While there may be many uncertainties in the assumptions made from manpower models, it should be appreciated that a bolder approach would allow more flexibility in planning,

and encourage delegation, rather than both over-treatment and under-utiliz-
ation of valuable dental manpower.

A cautious approach to change ?

(Bronkhorst, Truin, Klabbers, Plasschaert) The general argument for a reduction in dental manpower at the dental practitioner level is, therefore, strong,
but in individual countries the evaluation of future treatment needs has
proved arduous and the necessary adjustments in manpower difficult to
balance. The Dutch experience illustrates this. During the past decades the
imbalance between demand and supply of dental health care in Holland has
been a matter of serious concern. Between 1983 and 1987, the Dutch government, in response to the growing unemployment of dentists, decided to
reduce the intake of dental students from 480 to 120 a year. This involved the
closing of three (out of five) dental schools. This policy exemplifies planning
for short-term goals, yet it has long-term implications.

To investigate the matter, a computer simulation model of the supply and
demand characteristics of the dental health care system in the Netherlands
has been developed. The simulation includes major demographic, pathological, psychological, sociological and economic processes on the demand side;
while the availability of dentists, dental hygienists and factors that determine
their productivity are on the supply side. It can be used to study a wide variety
of policy options related to major aspects of the system for up to 40 years
ahead, thereby assisting in programme and policy planning.

The model suggests that despite an improvement in the oral health of
young people, the Dutch population in the year 2000 will have about 100
million restorations and 10 million cavities; about a quarter of the population
will be edentulous. The prediction is that there will be an annual need for
about an 8.5 million hours of dental work, which means that about 5000
dentists will be required in full-time employment. Taking into account the
structure of the Dutch population of dentists, and in order to avoid a shortage
of dentists, the study shows that the intake of dental students should actually
increase in 1995 from 120 to 180 students per year.

Not least because of the anomalies implied by experience in countries like
Holland, there are those who counsel caution in plans for radical change in
dental manpower in developed countries. *(Adatia)* In particular, public
attitudes to health can change again, or the demand for corrective measures
in an environment of longer life expectancy may prove larger than has been
projected from the current level of utilization of dental services.

(Gordon) For some, changing the clinical, technological and interventionist prescribing patterns of general dental practitioners is seen as fraught
with structural difficulties that are not going to be solved by a programme of
continuing education, mandatory or otherwise. This viewpoint is in clear

opposition to the optimistic one portrayed in the contribution on p. 70. The reasoning behind this contradiction in part concerns the nature of a 'profession'. Conventionally, it is argued, a profession is distinguished from other occupations by its service orientation. This assumes that dentists generally rely on accepted scientific standards rather than individual ones; that they restrict their work to the limits of their own technical competence; and that they put the patients' interests before their own. However, the clinical attitudes of what are largely self-employed dental practitioners differ substantially from those of the formal spokespersons for the profession, who are reputedly the models of proper clinical behaviour, and they are often at variance with the values of those who work in teaching institutions. Some explanation for this difference appears to lie in the reality of professional self-regulation. Fundamental to this reality is the question of whether a dentist is colleague-controlled or patient-controlled.

Independent practising dentists use general principles to deal with individual problems, whereas scientists investigate data in order to test, elaborate or arrive at general principles. There has and always will be an overwhelming bias, when applying science in general practice, to focus on mechanistic solutions and even occasionally to effect a treatment rather than not, irrespective of the existence of reliable knowledge about its precise outcome. Such an approach appears to be dissociated from the method by which the practitioner is paid.

Practitioners thus have an aim based upon action rather than knowledge *per se*. Successful action is preferred, but action with very little chance of success is preferred over no action at all. And the practitioner is most likely to believe that what he or she is doing is in the best interest of the patient. This has some considerable implications for the developing philosophies concerning minimum intervention (*see* p. 27). The practitioner also tends to be a pragmatist when defining needs and dental fitness, and is prone to rely on patient demand rather than on rigid legislation, with a strong instinct to trust the accumulation of knowledge based on personal experience.

It is as well to ponder over this 'dissenting voice', but few would dispute that *(Sheiham)* it is dentists with a broad education and training (*see* p. 77), and sensitive to community and individual needs and wants, who will be needed to work in the future integrated primary health care system. While future patterns of dental care will challenge their intellectual and professional skills, dentists will undoubtedly fulfil their roles as essential members of the health care team even though this will require many changes in dental education.

THE FUTURE MANAGEMENT OF ORAL DISEASES

(Pindborg) That the scope of dentistry reaches beyond the dental arches has

been strongly reflected in the dental literature of the past three decades. Diseases of the jaws, including the mandibular joints, the salivary glands and the oral mucosa, are now in the focus of dental research and dental practice. Diseases of the oral mucosa have for some time been in the foreground, particularly in relation to precancerous lesions and their association with different types of tobacco usage. It is surely mandatory that the dental curriculum and postgraduate training should change in the direction of more thorough teaching in these subjects.

(Johnson) Traditionally, in the West, intervention in oral health care has been mostly by professionally and expensively trained personnel. And at the community level, such care, whether in terms of health education (the effects of which are difficult to evaluate) or of active intervention (c.g. water fluoridation), has been aimed at all members of society, irrespective of the degree of risk. As argued in Chapter 2, these methods have not met with universal success and some have certainly been expensive. Even so, water fluoridation should remain as a pillar of preventive policy, where its implementation is politically and legally acceptable. On the other hand it should be remembered that defluoridation of local water supplies remains an equally important need in the many places where fluorosis is endemic.

In the future there might also be a place for legislative initiatives aimed at combating oral diseases. These could encompass the placing of taxes on, for example, sugar and tobacco; and advertising restrictions and health warnings on potentially dangerous products, such as high sucrose-containing foodstuffs and tobacco.

Screening for risk groups

It has been explained in Chapter 3 that caries and the periodontal diseases are best approached as conditions for which different individuals have very different degrees of risk. It is therefore irrational, and not cost-effective, to attempt literally to 'force down the throats' of every member of society the same preventive measures irrespective of their degree of risk. Apart from what may be regarded as uncontroversial general health education on diet and personal hygiene, evidence for the effectiveness of mass preventive intervention is, perhaps, strong for dental caries in Western societies (because of the widespread use of fluorides in various forms); indeterminate for oral cancer (there have been successes in a few intensive and expensive intervention programmes in high-risk communities such as in the Indian subcontinent); and neglible for destructive periodontitis. When it comes to professionally administered preventive measures – scale and polish, topical fluorides, even fissure sealants to list the most obvious – there must be the danger of over-treating the majority to reach the minority. It follows that decisions need to be made to move the dental profession away from attempting to 'treat' all members of society, in favour of establishing screening programmes so that a rational treatment and preventive strategy can be focused on those most in need. This should be less interventionist and more cost-effective; there are many precedents, such as screening for cervical cancer, and for risk factors in coronary heart disease and diabetes.

Approaches here could be based on sociological and demographic evidence: for example, the known predilection of certain socio-economic or immigrant populations for a high prevalence of dental caries or the known existence of a cultural risk factor, such as chewing tobacco or 'reverse smoking' in relation to oral cancer. Much of the screening might be done at less cost by appropriately trained ancillary staff. By this means, clinical observations and the taking of samples for biological tests, such as microbial 'counts', would become cheap and simple low-tech activities – even though their development may require expensive research. A community basis for laboratory investigations could also be encouraged.

Cancer is the most important oral mucosal disease because of its high morbidity and mortality. In most Western countries, squamous cell carcinoma of the oral mucous membrane accounts for some 1–3 per cent of all malignancies, with an incidence rate of some 4 per 100 000 per annum. In the whole of the Indian subcontinent and much of South East Asia, parts of South America and some Pacific islands, the incidence is up to 10 times as great. These high-prevalence geographical areas are largely explained by cultural practices, in particular the use of areca (betel) nut and smokeless tobacco; nutritional, genetic and socio-economic factors also probably play a part.

Detection of those at high risk of developing oral cancer is a high priority for the future and is possible to a considerable extent. In high-prevalence parts of the world the majority of oral carcinomas develop in relation to a pre-existing 'premalignant' lesion. Such lesions can be detected by clinical examination; and intervention programmes based on clinical screening and on advice to eliminate known aetiological factors have proved extremely successful in several carefully conducted studies, notably those in Sri Lanka[51] and in Southern India.[52]

Research into the aetiology, host resistance factors and pathogenesis of oral cancer and precancer is also advancing in many laboratories worldwide. The role of parasitic, fungal, bacterial and viral infections is becoming better understood, as is the role of the host immune system in modifying the progress of the lesion. A variety of laboratory methods can be used for assessing the probability of a premalignant lesion progressing to malignancy and for assessing the prognosis of a carcinoma. These include analysis of tissue structure, chromosomal and nuclear abnormalities, oncogene expression and activation, growth and abnormalities of cell proliferation, and the presence and expression of viral genome in cells. Many of these are as yet in the realm of research and not applicable to routine or chairside screening, but it is possible that, in the future, patients at risk may be identified by laboratory assay for infectious and immune status.

Vaccination

Progress towards the development of a safe and effective anti-caries vaccine continues[53] and knowledge about the relevant virulence factors of oral cariogenic micro-organisms grows. It has been established in principle that vaccination against caries is now feasible. However, the falling prevalence of caries in Western countries has removed some of the urgency there, and vaccine research is not receiving the same priority in research funding as it once did. However, some argue that there remains a need for such a vaccine for use in the high-risk groups in Western communities and, if a cost-effective way could be made to deliver it, for most members of society in many developing countries. Effective vaccination against one or more of the severe periodontal diseases is some distance away in the future.

Change and the individual

Individuals can often be readily motivated and educated to monitor aspects of their own general health. Clearly, in this activity, a balance needs to be struck at a level short of the paranoid; self-palpation of the breast for the possibility of cancer exemplifies both the possibilities and the problems of self-screening. Obviously, parents have a special educational role with their infants and younger children. There is no doubt that intelligent and motivated adults can make useful clinical observations, and diagnostic kits for home use are proliferating in the medical field. Such kits should be encouraged in dentistry but not until their validity, reliability, sensitivity and specificity are thoroughly established; here lie exciting challenges for clinical and laboratory research. Decisions should be made to devote a decent proportion of each nation's health budgets to such research which is, by its nature, both 'basic' and 'applied'.

Change and the professional

To encapsulate what has been said before, the priorities for dental professional personnel should be inverted from their traditional, medium-tech (*see* p. 78) treatment orientation to:

— counselling in matters of diet, hygiene and self-assessment;

— screening by clinical and laboratory/chairside tests;

— targeted prevention and minimal intervention;

— complex treatment.

TOWARDS ERADICATION OF MAJOR DISEASE

The foregoing account has given a broad perspective of future trends and needs. In this section, the future control of periodontal diseases and caries is considered in greater detail.

Periodontal diseases

(*Cutress*) Before it was understood that bacterial dental plaque is of prime aetiological significance in periodontal diseases, clinical treatments were essentially empirical. Two decades later, these empirical treatments still tend to dominate the approach to periodontal care. But, as described in Chapter 3, most chronic periodontal diseases are largely preventable, and established disease can usually be adequately controlled, except in high-risk individuals.

As with other therapies, periodontal care can be classified, in order of priority, as *primary* – to prevent the onset of diseases; *secondary* – to reverse or contain diseases; and *tertiary* – to prevent tooth loss from diseases. Clinical and epidemiological evidence increasingly supports this order of priority as the most appropriate and most cost-effective basis for management of the diseases and thus for improving oral health care for individuals and populations in the future. Primary prevention is best implemented through social/behavioural learning; it is basic to all periodontal care. Secondary prevention falls within the responsibility of auxiliary staff and the practitioner; whereas tertiary prevention is the responsibility of the auxiliary, practitioner and specialist.

Modern clinical and epidemiological findings on periodontal care counsel a conservative approach to treatment, with most emphasis and resources being directed towards primary prevention and least towards tertiary prevention. And with the limitations of current knowledge, prevention should, at least in the short term, continue to be based on the assumption of a non-specific effect of plaque. Plaque accumulation is modified by calculus and anatomical irregularities as well as by dietary, physiological and iatrogenic factors. Control of disease is aimed at reducing plaque levels and so improving the positive balance towards a healthy oral environment.

(*Holmgren*) There is, however, generally a paucity of information about the time required for the provision of periodontal treatment, especially in relation to the specific problems found in developing countries. One study has sought to determine the time required to provide oral hygiene and scaling in Chinese adults in Hong Kong, and to assess the effect on scaling time when this procedure was deferred until six months after comprehensive oral hygiene instruction. Preliminary results indicate that the oral hygiene instruction took an average of over 40 minutes and scaling provided during this initial phase of treatment required a mean of 26 minutes per sextant. When initial scaling was deferred until six months after oral hygiene instruction, the mean time for scaling was reduced to only 12 minutes per sextant.

High-risk groups. (Johnson) Of the high-risk groups in the population susceptible to the development of destructive periodontitis, a very small proportion can be explained on the basis of having an intercurrent systemic disease or a defect of host defence. Screening for such conditions is thus unlikely to be practicable on a community basis, but must form part of the assessment of patients who have severe periodontal breakdown. In the immediate future, population screening may best be approached clinically – by identifying those with 'severe disease for age'; the CPITN (*see* Chapter 3), will facilitate this. Such screening can be carried out in institutions, schools and places of work; and in the armed services and similar 'captive' groups – it should certainly be performed routinely in dental clinics. 'Susceptible' individuals need then to be referred for full oral and general health 'work up'.

Research aimed at developing laboratory markers of disease susceptibility and activity, which might be applied to blood, saliva, subgingival plaque or gingival crevicular fluid (*see* Chapter 3), is making rapid progress around the world, and is likely to make a large contribution to the management of periodontal diseases in the future.

Caries and restorations

(Tala) Further dramatic changes will be seen over the next few decades, and enthusiastic adoption of today's health promotion messages will significantly increase dental health. This is nothing new, for dentists have generally succeeded in bringing up their own children with totally sound teeth and no fillings. *(Hooper)* There is also good evidence that restorations in dentists' mouths last considerably longer than has been reported in studies of general populations. When the dental treatment received by a group of dentists during their student days and since qualification was examined in an attempt to determine whether or not these individuals had succeeded in maintaining an especially favourable restorative status, it was found that half of the restorations had lasted at least 15 years or were continuing to function. Dentists presumably practice prevention in their own mouths, and their professional knowledge ensures that only restorations of high quality are undertaken. They are also very careful to ensure that restorations are only replaced when this is unavoidable. It may be that dentists' (and their

families') needs for treatment now forebode the dental treatment needs of adults in general in the future.

(Tala) It is pertinent to ask whether caries could actually be eradicated among all children and young people by deployment of the effective and economic (but as yet little used) methods for prevention that have been available for several decades (*see* Chapter 2). There is good evidence that the answer is 'yes'. For example, in a rural health centre in central Finland a preventive oral health care philosophy was introduced 15 years ago. The mean index of decayed, missing and filled teeth among 12-year-olds was around 10 at the beginning of the programme; today it is 0.8. The estimate for 25-year-olds in the year 2000 is that there will be an index value of around 2 compared with today's score of 15. Thus children and young adults may need very little restorative intervention for caries if all the possibilities of modern prevention are utilized.

(Anusavice) One of the major problems that the dental profession will encounter in any future quest to achieve widespread acceptance of a preventive approach to dental care is the failure of insurance plans and other third-party funding bodies, administrators of public dental care services, educators and the public to overturn the traditional belief that restorations eliminate caries. This belief is likely to persist even in the face of the compelling evidence that restorative treatment rather easily begets more restorative treatment (*see* Chapter 3). Coupled to this shortsightedness is the failure of the dental profession to demand compensation for preventive therapy and for counselling sessions with patients so that they can demonstrate the benefits and tooth-conservation potential of this approach.

To encourage practitioners to adopt a preventive approach rather than to adhere to the more aggressive philosophy which suggests 'when in doubt, drill and fill to eliminate disease' it was concluded at the symposium *Criteria for Placement and Replacement of Dental Restorations* [15] that:

Professional remuneration should be based on comprehensive care, recognizing professional time and services rendered for the purpose of conserving and optimizing the longevity of the patient's dentition. Remuneration should not be based on technical services alone.

While caries clearly is a major cause of restoration failure, many restorations are replaced because of the quality of the marginal area (*see* p. 25) with no conclusive evidence of active caries. It is obvious that this deep-seated compulsion to replace defective restorations rather than to diagnose accurately and treat the true disease state will not be easily overcome in the near future, especially in much of the Western world. As an interim measure, a system for standardization of restoration quality combined with an assessment of caries risk should be adopted. The quality evaluation system of the California Dental Association provides a potential model for establishing preventive criteria, restorative criteria, and for evaluating the quality of treatment plans. It can also serve as a useful standard for self and peer evaluation of the overall quality of dental care. However, this system must be supplemented with criteria for evaluation of the patient's current caries risk and the likely success in shifting him or her to a lower risk level.

THE FUTURE FOR ORTHODONTICS

One of the urgent future requirements in orthodontics, the need for methods of objective assessment of treatment needs and risk, has already been discussed (see Chapter 3). But the very role of the general dental practitioner in the future practice of orthodontics is also of pressing importance.

(Stephens) The recently improved dental health in most Western countries means that orthodontic treatment is now potentially relevant for a larger proportion of the child population. It is also increasingly relevant to areas of adult dental practice. These factors, together with the adoption of a more preventive approach to dental care, have made many general dental practitioners aware that orthodontics is an area of practice they can no longer afford to ignore. Orthodontic courses are much in demand and there are requests from undergraduates to improve their training in orthodontics. However, as discussed earlier, there are limits both to the proportion of children (and adults) who are prepared to undergo orthodontic treatment and to those who can truly be said to benefit from it. If both under- and over-treatment of malocclusions are to be avoided, the questions that require answers are: which malocclusions should be treated? – and how much of this treatment should be provided by the non-specialist?

Why, indeed, does the general practitioner need to be involved at all? Some take the view that since a majority of orthodontic treatment should ideally be carried out by specialists, then less time should be given to orthodontic teaching at the undergraduate level in order to allow dental schools to concentrate their resources on producing a greater number of fully trained postgraduate specialists.[54] On the other hand, there is no real evidence that a formal specialist training is essential for excellence in orthodontic treatment: a more moderate majority thus take the view that the general dental practitioner should continue to play a key role in the recognition of malocclusion and in the initiation of simple interceptive measures for the foreseeable future. They also point out that as specialists tend to be concentrated in areas of dense population, so general practitioners working in more sparsely inhabited regions will need to have more in the way of orthodontic skills.

A failure of traditional orthodontic departments to provide adequate undergraduate training in some parts of the USA in the past caused many dentists to seek 'motel' orthodontic courses. This backlash has led to friction between the specialist and non-specialist: the orthodontist feels that hard-won skills are being set at naught, while generalists see their clinical competence being called into question. Inadequate undergraduate orthodontic training may also have adverse effects on the overall standard of orthodontic care in other ways. There is some evidence to show that the greater the effort put into undergraduate education, the more selective graduates will be in the cases they are prepared to treat when in independent practice, and the greater will be the proportion that they feel should be referred for specialist treatment. This North American research also suggests that graduates who have received little orthodontic instruction perceive orthodontists as holding back on straightforward information, whilst those who have been trained more extensively as undergraduates are generally satisfied with the role the specialist plays.

If it is accepted that the general practitioner will continue to play a role in the provision of orthodontic care, there seem to be three steps which must be taken by those responsible for administering dental education :

–   The role of the practitioner must be carefully defined and the licensing authority must ensure that the graduates of each school qualify with at least the minimum skills necessary to ensure that this role can be fulfilled.

–   Adequate postgraduate practitioner training should be available.

–   There should be an appropriate number of identifiable and highly trained orthodontic specialists to accept patients whose treatment falls outside the skills of the referring practitioner, i.e., there should be an indicative specialist register.

At the inception of the British NHS, provision was made for a state-funded orthodontic consultant service, which the practitioner could use for advice without charge – and this has been shown to be effective. However, recent growth in demand has meant that the consultant service is now overstretched in most areas, and patients may have to wait many months for such advice. The outcome has been that only a small proportion of practitioner patients are so referred. Fortunately, the advent of the microcomputer should mean that, in the near future, expert advice will be immediately available in the surgery from computer-based systems.[55]

THE FUTURE FOR ORAL HEALTH IN DEVELOPING COUNTRIES

(Barmes) At least in relation to dental and periodontal diseases, the reader may expect a different set of predictions and suggestions for the developing countries than have been advanced so far. Strangely enough, this is not the case. Although the rise and fall of dental caries occurred in various European, North American and South Pacific industrialized countries over various

periods, at various rates and to various peaks, the major part of the cycle seems to have taken 100 years or more (Figure facing p. 1). By contrast, it has now been observed in countries like Singapore, Hong Kong, and more recently, Japan, that the cycle can occur over a period of 40 years. The figures point to there being countries which experience little more than a minor 'blip' on the curve with others experiencing only a moderate rise and fall over 20 –40 years. Their experience of caries rises to levels little different from those that industrialized countries are reaching towards the ends of their cycles. Peoples already seriously affected will return to more or less where they began, by 2025 or possibly before. Indeed, it can be predicted that what applies to the industrialized countries in 2025 will also be appropriate for countries at every level of development by that time.

Planning dental care for populations

(Pinto) In non-developed countries (*per capita* income up to US$ 1000), where disease rates are tending to rise (*see* Chapter 2), a major challenge facing dentistry is therefore to prevent, over the next few decades, populations from being burdened with an increasing incidence of dental caries as economic development takes place. The future can only be built on what is done today. There is clearly an immediate need for mass community preventive measures, but these require careful planning. By definition, planning involves deliberate intervention in the course of events. It acts through the selection of groups or sectors to be benefitted, emphasizing certain forms of progress with the necessary authority to solve conflicts and thereby to effectively develop the proposed plan. It is worth stressing that plans governing actions are the ones that are effected; not those that are simply thought about.

It is impossible and irrelevant for poor communities, burdened by high levels of the disease, to adopt the responses of the developed world, since it is necessary to reduce *at once* the existing large volume of dental problems and not to wait for solutions embedded in an uncertain process of economic growth. This is not a new problem, it having been brought clearly into discussion globally for at least 10 years. But action has been slow; most public health programmes have covered only small populations and any research, some of which is of doubtful relevance, has been done mainly by richer countries where the necessary facilities exist.

The following scheme may be put forward for implementation in the short and medium term in the non-industrialized world.

— Dental activities should be planned for the population at large; pilot projects should gradually be substituted by comprehensive programmes. (This approach is illustrated by examples from specific countries in Chapter 4).

—   The main thrust should be concentrated on priority groups as determined on economic grounds and by epidemiological methods; and
coverage of such groups with primary dental care, irrespective of
financial, ethnic, religious or political constraints, should be as complete as possible. Where there is a large low-income population,
neither the market-led model nor the indirect rendering of services
(*see* p. 9) are advisable if the goal of the country is to reduce the levels
of the disease.

—   The implementation of preventive and educational programmes
should be the main line of action. These should be started at once,
without waiting for well-structured health systems or dependable
treatment-based service networks. But great care must be taken to
select appropriate methods. In developing countries, bringing
together the necessary conditions for a preventive method to be
effective is a difficult task. For example, fluoride mouthrinsing in
schools and salt fluoridation, both excellent in principle, have met
with only limited success in Brazil for various infrastructural and
social reasons. It has therefore been decided that water fluoridation
and yearly or semi-annual applications of acidulated phosphate fluoride gel are more appropriate for reducing the levels of dental caries
there, at least in the middle term.

—   Prevention of infection and cross-infection in dental practice should
be stressed, because of the severity of conditions such as hepatitis and
AIDS, even though this has economic implications.

—   Specific research into oral health at the community level should be
undertaken. There is a need for short-term financial resources, including those from international bodies, to enable experienced research workers in preventive and social dentistry to deploy their
talents in developing countries (*see* the FINNIDA scheme in Tanzania; p. 61). They would provide the necessary information for planning
and effecting health care models for use in local programmes. Effort
at the international level would be aimed at building regional planning
and programming models and making them available to countries for
use in local service units as appropriate. By the end of this century the
developing world should be prepared to control its own oral health
problems.

Future dental education in the developing world

(*Johnson*) Too many developing countries have established dental schools
with curricula modelled on the Western pattern, with their emphasis on
treatment and high technology. A more appropriate curriculum, as discussed

on p. 62, needs a strong foundation of the basic and the medical sciences, with relevant epidemiology and community health. Strong emphasis should be placed on the training of ancillaries capable of the screening, educative and minimal intervention strategies outlined above. Close liaison needs to be maintained between Ministries of Health and Ministries of Education. The part to be played by oral health strategies as catalysts for improvements in general health is increasingly recognized. This attitude is summed up in the World Health Organization slogan *Health through Oral Health*, and has been well argued at an earlier symposium.[56]

All this provides the dental profession with an opportunity to lead. The rapid growth in scientific knowledge of oral diseases, the interesting changes in disease prevalence and distribution and the continued improvement in world communication combine to make this an exciting time in dentistry. Cutbacks in teaching, research and clinical opportunities in the West are matched by increasing needs and opportunities in developing countries. From a global perspective, the challenges and opportunities are immense.

CONCLUSIONS

(Pinto) Moving from piecemeal dental treatment towards oral health is a long-term process that clearly requires some painful discussion on the future roles of dentists and other oral health workers. There is no universally accepted, comprehensive model to copy, and, at the moment, it seems as if tradition is guiding the educational and care delivery system rather more than any systematic effort to apply the results of research and common sense. The pessimistic view is that the present philosophy in oral health care in developed countries will continue. This could well lead to chaos with thousands of dentists becoming unemployed and still the populations being without proper oral health care services.

It is very clear that the production of dentists and any other mainly clinical oral health personnel has never been sufficient, alone, to solve the problem of oral and dental diseases. A successful approach to oral health problems requires adequate legislation, appropriate planning, comprehensive implementation and meticulous monitoring and evaluation. A reliable and flexible information system is thus essential; and the main emphasis should be on health promotion and prevention, with restorative and rehabilitative services playing a complementary role.

(Lester) It is rather easy to mouth fervid generalities concerning the way things will or will not be, or what the profession must or must not do. Most would agree that epidemiological analysis is fundamental to a proper predictive approach. There is a problem, however, in that many in the profession can only engage in day-to-day crisis management because the tools and authority for forward decision-making are simply not theirs to apply; political

and economic factors, both local and global, may well exert the stronger influence.[57] Nevertheless, it is unintelligent not to try to predict and then try to adapt as well as possible.[58]

The way forward would seem to be through less mechanical, more scientifically based, more sensitive and happy-to-be-conservative dentists. The present generation has been trained (and is training others) to provide *things* for *patients*: but dental personnel should aim and be happy to influence communities and the oral environments of their members with minimal invasive interference. The challenge will be to continue to impart the skills and, at the same time, encourage both the appropriate attitudinal change and the creation of a reward system for reinforcing this preferred behaviour. Perhaps the most important challenge of our times in oral health care is the matching of health services to the prevailing epidemiological features and typical problems of the society in question.

6
Summary

It is a common notion that freedom from oral and dental diseases can be achieved through an invasive restorative approach, and such an approach is strong in many parts of the world. However, improved understanding of the consequences and shortfalls of restorative treatment as a method of achieving oral health in populations endorses the concept that prevention, supported by health promotion and education, should be the foundation for oral health if it is to be successful on a large scale both in the developing world and in industrialized (and post-industrialized) countries. The changing picture of the epidemiology and natural history of caries and periodontal diseases strengthens this view.

It is possible to forecast that dentists, in addition to becoming increasingly concerned with promoting oral health at the community level, will become more specifically concerned with the care of patients who have:

— important systemic conditions (including HIV infection);

— particular high-risk susceptibility to caries or periodontal diseases;

— relatively rare oral conditions;

— complex restorative needs;

— certain significant occlusal disorders.

Indeed, it has been predicted that within the working lifetimes of some present members of the profession, dentists will become more like oral physicians and will work with a variety of auxiliaries in the endeavour to bring about maximum oral health for populations. It seems that countries with comprehensive dental services will have to prepare themselves for a gradual change to a situation in which the rather common invasive treatment of today is a much less frequent occurrence.

The uncertain relevance of today's dentistry to the oral health issues of tomorrow raises some fundamental questions. Much of the teaching in undergraduate dental schools reflects yesterday's requirements. One consequence is that the training of dentists has been concentrated on surgical treatment procedures as opposed to the preventive and communication tasks which are needed on a large scale. At the same time, many dentists have not been prepared for the relatively complex diagnostic and treatment tasks that are likely to confront them in the next few decades. There is a need for a fundamental reappraisal of dental education. Initiative and innovation are required now in order to bring about fundamental changes to suit it to the needs of the changing world. There is a clear need for all those involved with the provision of oral health care, especially licensing bodies and those responsible for health care delivery, to widen their perceptions of the issues at stake and thereby enable forward-looking curriculum development.

Appendix

The following summary statements, first published in the *British Dental Journal*,[59] were compiled from the invited presentations and from the subsequent discussion at the conference.

1   Background

1.1   It is recognized that in most industrialized countries there has been a dramatic reduction in recent years in the prevalence and extent of some oral diseases, notably dental caries. The wide use of fluorides, particularly in the form of toothpaste, is thought to be largely responsible. At the same time, more people are retaining their natural teeth longer and aspiring to maintain a functional and aesthetic dentition throughout life. This, combined with ageing populations, has the potential to increase demands on some oral care services. By contrast, levels of caries in many developing parts of the world, which had until recently been low, are rising and the prevalence of the disease in these areas has exceeded or may soon exceed the levels now seen in industrialized countries. The main reason for this increase is believed to be altered dietary habits.

1.2   By encouraging oral health education and self-care in its various forms, and by eliminating diseased tissue and restoring function and aesthetics, the dental profession has made an important contribution to the improvements in oral health and well-being in many countries. However, there may be a potential for over-treatment where dentist-to-population ratios are high, while in areas where resources are scarce or poorly distributed, many people do not receive or demand adequate oral health care and many may experience unnecessary pain and tooth loss.

1.3   It is easy to believe that dental treatment automatically results in oral health. It is, therefore, not surprising that the traditional restorative approach has a strong influence on dental practice in many parts of the world. Yet, restorative treatment *per se* has been shown to have many shortcomings and does not, on its own, ensure oral health.

2   Management of dental caries

2.1   Today's greater understanding of the caries process and the improved potential for its prevention and control mean that it is possible for most people not to lose their dentitions as a result of this disease. This goal can be achieved through optimum use of fluoride, preventive self-care including an enlightened approach to sugar consumption, the use of techniques such as fissure sealants, and with restorative treatment as necessary. The present emphasis on a surgical approach to caries treatment should be limited to the minimum.

2.2 Fluoridation of the water supply remains a highly effective and economic means of reducing the prevalence of dental caries and, wherever possible, it should be used in areas with high caries experience. Other methods of distributing fluoride, especially through toothpaste, should also be used. Partial defluoridation should be effected in water supplies with excessive fluoride levels.

2.3 An assessment of susceptibility to, and risk of, caries should be an integral part of treatment planning and an essential precursor to any restorative treatment. But because caries is a multifactorial disease, assessments of susceptibility must themselves be multifactorial. Standard methods of diagnosis, both clinical and laboratory (including microbiological), have poor sensitivity and specificity, and criteria for the replacement of restorations are even more imprecise. Further research and training are required to improve diagnostic methods and standards.

2.4 Research should continue in an effort to develop more effective arresting and remineralizing agents for possible widespread clinical or home use. Further research is also required to determine the logistics of a preventive, non-invasive approach to dental caries management and to investigate the potential for minimizing the need for rotary instruments. In some parts of the world these are not readily available.

3   Management of periodontal diseases

3.1 Understanding of the nature and distribution of periodontal diseases has improved greatly over recent years. Severe destructive periodontal diseases are not as prevalent as had previously been thought, and there is controversy as to whether gingivitis and destructive forms of periodontitis have the same or differing aetiologies. The control of periodontal breakdown is possible in the majority of people using known and readily available methods involving oral hygiene and minimal professional treatment. It seems that these methods make it possible for most people to maintain adequate periodontal health and (together with effective caries control) a functioning dentition for life.

3.2 Further research is required to enable the early identification and treatment of those individuals who are susceptible to severe destructive periodontal diseases. The presence of severe disease relative to the person's age and oral hygiene is perhaps the best predictor at present. Special attention should be focused on juvenile periodontitis.

3.3 Periodontal screening in dental practice is facilitated by using a standardized procedure. The Community Periodontal Index of Treatment Needs (CPITN) method of recording levels of periodontal disease has been found to be useful and workable for this purpose and it is in widespread use.

4 Oral health care of patients with systemic diseases

4.1 Advances in medical practice in areas such as transplant surgery and in irradiation and drug therapy, together with the advent of HIV, have resulted in new populations of patients requiring special precautions during dental treatment. In some Western countries, there is growth in legal actions against dentists involving increasingly large financial settlements, many of which arise from failure to recognize the needs of medically compromised patients. Dentists also have an important role in the early diagnosis of systemic disease, including especially HIV infection; and all oral health care programmes should include active intervention aimed at the prevention, early diagnosis and treatment of the rarer but sometimes life-threatening diseases which affect the mouth, such as cancer. These and other factors combine to increase the importance that should be attached to dentists having a thorough knowledge of systemic diseases, including their oral manifestations and implications in oral health care.

4.2 Spread of the HIV infection in particular has caused a reassessment of cross-infection procedures in dental practice, which must be adequate to protect patients and staff. The provision of sufficient resources for this purpose should be a priority in all countries. This is recognized as a problem in the poorer parts of the world.

5 Management of malocclusion

5.1 There is little doubt that orthodontic treatment is highly desirable for individuals with severe malocclusion and for the treatment of certain congenital abnormalities. However, in some industrialized countries, the demand for treatment of mild malocclusion is very high and treatment, as currently practised, is frequently unsuccessful in the long term; and it may have little demonstrable health, social or psychological benefit. The use of public funds for the treatment of some mild malocclusions is questionable. The development of objective criteria to indicate the precise nature of deformities requiring treatment with a high probability of a successful outcome would be very beneficial.

5.2 Undergraduates should be trained sufficiently in orthodontics so that they can, as general dental practitioners, diagnose correctly and appreciate the limitations of orthodontic care in their hands. Further, they should appreciate the scope and limitations of specialist skills.

6 Implementation of oral health care services

6.1 The knowledge and expertise to implement effective, economic and appropriate oral health care services exist, but the mechanisms required for integrating the science of oral care within the service infrastructure are generally lacking. In order to improve overall the oral health in a country, oral health care services should be planned in full knowledge of the oral health situation of the whole population and be accommodated within the context of the prevailing social, epidemiological and political conditions. This implies a public health approach. While services should be properly distributed geographically, they should also be targeted to meet locally identified needs and demands. Full integration of oral and general health care services appears to be the most optimistic way forwards, with effective involvement of school teachers, parents and general health workers.

6.2 Prevention supported by health promotion and education should be the foundation for oral health if it is to be successful on a large scale in both developing areas of the world and in industrialized countries. It is believed that preventive programmes in oral health integrated with primary health care offer the best possibilities for this in affluent as well as in poorer rural areas of the world, although there is a need for further community-based research in this area.

6.3 While both the industrialized and the developing countries have an opportunity and a duty to encourage mutual sharing of experiences, there is no substitute for the development of local expertise in each country. The adoption of the existing Western pattern of oral health care services is not necessarily appropriate for developing countries. Rather, all countries should be encouraged to seek practical and realistic programmes tailored to their own needs.

6.4 Emphasis upon preserving a strategic functioning part of the remaining dentition, rather than the meticulous restoration of what is damaged or missing, should be seen as desirable aims in the management of patients who have experienced gross oral disease. There may be an increasing need for some relatively complex restorative treatments. However, oral health care for older people may, overall, require less restorative treatment than is often thought to be the case, though the psychological benefits of such treatment should be given proper consideration.

6.5 In industrialized countries, existing public and social insurance schemes generally reward those who intervene and provide treatment. Methods of remuneration must be found which encourage continuing care and non-invasive preventive techniques.

6.6 Comprehensive monitoring and evaluation systems are necessary in all countries, with effective feedback to planners and to field workers. Adjustments should then be made, as necessary, according to the objectives of the service and in the light of the realities of everyday living and current disease levels.

7 Personnel

7.1 A rational oral health personnel policy avoiding both gross over-supply and serious shortage should be an important goal for all countries. Such a policy should aim to ensure an equitable distribution of services for the whole population. However, as personnel predictions are particularly subject to inaccuracy, realistic options for future development should be kept flexible and reviewed regularly.

7.2 In industrialized countries, the reductions in the prevalence of oral diseases and improvements in oral health care will, if sustained, result in a future need for fewer dentists than previously expected. However, if oral health and care are to be widespread, dentists will have to accept responsibility both for health counselling on a community scale and for oral disease management in patients who may tend to have increasingly complex diagnostic and care problems. In those parts of the world where oral disease levels are rising, emphasis on health promotion at the community level is likely to offset the need for substantially more dentists than at present.

7.3 Opinions differ as to the desirable balance between different categories of oral health care workers, and each country should seek solutions appropriate to its circumstances. However, it seems that much of the care required in implementing preventive health care programmes could be provided by auxiliaries and other primary health care workers. The demand for multi-purpose auxiliary personnel is likely to rise, especially in developing countries. In addition to a shortage of resources and personnel, a problem in many of these countries is the maldistribution of existing manpower, which is largely confined to serving the middle-class populations in the cities. This frequently follows because training has been undertaken mainly in an urban setting.

7.4 It has been predicted that within the working lifetimes of some present members of the profession, dentists will become more like oral physicians and will work with a variety of auxiliary personnel in the endeavour to bring about maximum oral health for populations, though concentrating upon those who have been identified as being especially susceptible (at high risk) to caries or periodontal diseases.

8   Education

8.1   Much of the teaching in undergraduate dental schools reflects yesterday's requirements. One consequence of this is that the training of dentists has been concentrated on surgical treatment procedures as opposed to the preventive and communication tasks which are needed on a large scale. At the same time, many dentists have not been prepared for the relatively complex diagnostic and treatment tasks that are likely to confront them in the next few decades. There is a need for a fundamental reappraisal of dental education. Initiative and innovation are required now in order to bring about fundamental changes to suit it to the needs of the changing world. The undergraduate curriculum should be reviewed to achieve a better balance between theoretical knowledge of the basic sciences and their clinical applications; and greater prominence should be placed upon the control of disease processes.

8.2   There is a danger that a forward-looking undergraduate curriculum may conflict with current arrangements for the provision of services and with current guidelines issued by licensing authorities. To enhance the possibilities for imaginative innovation, a radical approach is required to encourage coherent change, and over a wide geographic front. The development of dental training and services should take place at a rate commensurate with the development of public knowledge and attitudes towards oral health and care. Account should also be taken of the fact that many undergraduate dental students at present have a prior expectation of doing what dentists have traditionally done; they want to learn surgery (and orthodontics), not prevention and counselling. Questions remain as to how university teaching staff can be brought fully up-to-date so as to assist the change in emphasis towards prevention. However, this requirement has to be reconciled with the need to teach technically excellent restorative work. Interventional techniques have to be taught, yet the mere fact that they are taught means that they rather easily come to form the basis of teaching and of subsequent practice.

8.3   In general, though with notable exceptions, it seems that undergraduate education in orthodontics, as with other aspects of dentistry, is inadequate and fails to provide an acceptable basis for accurate diagnostic skills and understanding of the prognosis of treatment outcomes.

8.4   In a period of rapid change it is essential that effective mechanisms are established for regular updating of knowledge and techniques.

Research into the most effective methods of postgraduate education would seem to be a priority. Formal systems of relicensing may have worthwhile benefits.

9 The future

9.1 A fundamental issue facing dentistry and oral health care is the relevance of current practices to the needs of the future. There are many challenges, and these differ according to the circumstances and histories of each country. An immediate issue for developing countries is the prevention of any further increase in the prevalence of oral diseases and the provision of emergency care to their entire populations. Countries with comprehensive dental services will have to prepare themselves for a gradual change to a situation, within 40 years from now, when the rather common invasive treatment of today is a much less frequent occurrence. In bringing about these changes, cohesion within the profession will be essential, especially when such burning questions are being asked as: 'What practical steps should be taken now?' and: 'How can people be educated to the need to pay, directly or indirectly, for prevention?'

9.2 There is a clear need for all those involved with the provision of oral health care, especially licensing bodies and those responsible for health care delivery, to widen their perceptions of the issues at stake and thereby enable forward-looking curriculum development. It was agreed that the recommendations concerning the need for change in the undergraduate curriculum should be sent to every national dental council involved with dental curricula, with a plea for urgent consideration of the issues raised during the conference.

References

1. Cutress TW, Ainamo J, Sardo Infirri J. The CPITN procedure for identifying periodontal treatment needs in individuals and populations. *Int Dent J* 1987; **37**: 222–33.
2. Epidemiology, etiology, and prevention of periodontal diseases. Technical Report Series No. 621. Geneva: World Health Organization, 1978.
3. Pilot T. Implementation of preventive periodontal programs at the community level. *In* Frandsen A. (ed). *Public health aspects of periodontal disease*. Chicago: Quintessence, 1984.
4. Pilot T, Barmes D E. An update on periodontal conditions in adults measured by CPITN. *Int Dent J* 1987; **37**: 169–72.
5. Loe H, Ancrud A, Boysen A, Morrison E. Natural history of periodontal disease in man. Rapid, moderate and no loss of attachment in Sri Lankan labourers 14-46 years of age. *J Clin Perio* 1986; **13**: 431–40.
6. Abdellatif H M, Burt B A. An epidemiological investigation into the relative importance of age and oral hygiene status as determinants of periodontitis. *J Dent Res* 1987; **66**: 13–8.
7. Nabers C L, Stalker W H, Esparza D, Naylor B, Canales S. Tooth loss in 1535 treated periodontal patients. *J Perio* 1988; **59**: 297–300.
8. Genco R J, Christersson L A, Zambon J J. Juvenile periodontitis. *Int Den J* 1986; **36**: 168–76.
9. Kornman K S. Nature of periodontal diseases; assessment of diagnosis. *J Perio Res* 1987; **22**: 192–204.
10. Zahradnik R T, Dankers I. Accuracy and reliability of chairside assay for sulcular neutral proteases. *J Dent Res* 1988; **67**: 328.
11. Moore W E C. Microbiology of periodontal disease. *J Perio Res* 1987; **22**: 335–41.
12. Downer M C. Changing patterns of disease in the Western World. *In* Guggenheim B (ed). *Cariology today.* pp 1–12. Basel: Karger, 1984.
13. Palmer J D, Pitter A F V. Differences in dental caries levels between 8-year old children in Bath from different socio-economic groups. *Comm Dent Health* 1988; **5**: 363–7.
14. Elderton R J. Implications of recent dental health services research on the future of operative dentistry. *J Publ Health Dent* 1985; **45**: 101–5.
15. Anusavice K J (ed). *Quality evaluation of dental restorations: Criteria for placement and replacement*. Chicago: Quintessence, 1989.
16. Elderton R J, Nuttall N M. Variation among dentists in planning treatment. *Br Dent J* 1983; **154**: 201–6.
17. Thylstrup A, Bille J, Grist V. Radiographic and observed tissue changes in approximal carious lesions at the time of operative treatment. *Caries Res* 1986; **20**: 75–84.
18. Benn D K, Watson D F. Correlation between film position, bitewing shadows, clinical pitfalls, and the histologic size of approximal lesions. *Quintessence Int* 1989; **20**: 131–41.

19. Carr L M. Dental health of children in Australia, 1977–1985. *Aust Dent J* 1988; **33**: 205–11.
20. Barmes D E. Indicators for oral health and their implications for industralized countries. *Int Dent J* 1983; **33**: 60–6.
21. National Health and Medical Research Council (1984). Safety of dental amalgam. *Aust Dent J* 1985; **30**: 131–2.
22. Elderton R J. Longitudinal study of dental treatment in the General Dental Service in Scotland. *Br Dent J* 1983; **155**: 91–6.
23. Craig G G. Towards a rational approach to topical fluoride therapy at the mixed dentition stage. *Int Dent J* 1981; **31**: 121–4.
24. Simonsen R J. Retention and effectiveness of a single application of white sealant after 10 years. *JADA* 1987; **115**: 31–6.
25. Handelman S L, Leverett D H, Espeland M A, Curzon J A. Clinical radiographic evaluation of sealed carious and sound tooth surfaces. *JADA* 1986; **113**: 751–4.
26. Craig G G, Powell K R, Cooper M H. Clinical appearance of permanent successors after nonextraction treatment of grossly carious primary molars in highly anxious children. *J Dent Child* 1987; **54**: 170–5.
27. Elderton R J. Preventively-orientated restorations and restorative procedures. *In* Elderton R J (ed). *Positive Dental Prevention*. pp.82–92. London: Heinemann Medical, 1987.
28. Knight G. The tunnel restoration. *Dent Outlook* 1984; **10**: 53–7.
29. Oral health surveys: Basic methods. (3rd edn.). Geneva: World Health Organization, 1987.
30. Prahl-Andersen B. The need for orthodontic treatment. *Angle Orthod* 1978; **48**: 1–9.
31. A guide to oral health epidemiological investigations. Geneva: World Health Organization, 1979.
32. Berg R. Post-retention analysis of treatment problems and failures in 264 consecutively treated cases. *Eur J Orthod* 1979; **1**: 55–68.
33. Elderton R J, Clark J D. Orthodontic treatment in the General Dental Service assessed by the Occlusal Index. *Br J Orthod* 1983; **10**: 178–86.
34. Greenspan D, Greenspan J S, Hearst NG et al. Relation of oral hairy leukoplakia to infection with the human immunodeficiency virus and the risk of developing AIDS. *J Infect Dis* 1987; **155**: 475–81.
35. Scully C, Elkom M. Lichen planus: review and update on pathogenesis. *J Oral Pathol* 1985; **14**: 431–58.
36. James J, Ferguson M M, Forsyth A, Tulloch N, Lamey P J. Oral lichenoid reactions related to mercury sensitivity. *Brit J Oral Max-Fac Surg* 1987; **25**: 474–80.
37. Hietanen J, Pihlman K, Forstrom L, Linder E, Reunala T. No evidence of hypersensitivity to dental restorative metals in oral lichen planus. *Scand J Dent Res* 1987; **95**: 320–27.
38. Lind P O. Oral lichenoid reactions related to composite restorations. *Acta Odont Scand* 1988; **46**: 63–5.
39. Editorial. Oral snuff; a preventable carcinogenic hazard. *Lancet* 1986; **ii**: 198–200.
40. World Health Organization. Alternative systems of oral care delivery. WHO Technical Report Series No 750. Geneva: World Health Organization, 1987.

41. Barmes D E, Tala H. Health manpower out of balance: conflicts and prospects for oral health. *In* Bankowski Z, Mejia A (eds). *Health manpower out of balance – Conflicts and prospects.* pp 158–67. Geneva: CIOMS, 1987.

42. Dental Strategy Review Group. *Towards better dental health - guidelines for the future.* London: HMSO, 1981.

43. Cm 249. *Promoting Better Health.* London: HMSO.

44. Coventry P, Holloway P J, Lennon M A, Mellor A C. A capitation system for the treatment of children in the General Dental Service. *Brit Dent J* 1985; **160**: 174–7.

45. Department of Health and Social Security. *Report of the Committee of Enquiry into Unnecessary Dental Treatment.* London: HMSO.

46. Sheiham A, Marmot M, Rawson D, Ruck N. Food values: Health and diet. *In* Jowell R, Witherspoon S, Brook L (eds). *British social attitudes.* The 1987 Report. pp 95–119. Aldershot: Gower, 1987.

47. Seow W K. Bottle caries: a challenge to preventive dentistry. *Dentistry Today* 1987; **3**: 1–9.

48. Allred H, Duckworth R, Johnson N W, Slack G L. Proposals for planned change in dental education and practice. *Br Dent J* 1972; **133**: 173–9.

49. Kirk EEJ. Changing disease patterns and social expectations in dentistry. *Ann R Aust Coll Dent Surg* 1984; **8**: 97–105.

50. Locker D. Measuring oral health: A conceptual framework. *Comm Dent Health* 1988; **5**: 3–18.

51. Warnakulasuriya K A A S, Ekanyake A N I, Sivayoham S A et al. Utilisation of primary health care workers for early detection of oral cancer and precancer cases in Sri Lanka. *Bull WHO* 1984; **62**: 243–250.

52. Gupta P C, Mehta F S, Pindborg J J et al. Intervention study for primary prevention of oral cancer among 36 000 Indian tobacco users. 1986; *Lancet* **i**: 1235–8.

53. Russell R R B, Johnson N W. The prospects for vaccination against dental caries. *Br Dent J* 1987; **162**: 29–34.

54. Shaw W C. Improving British orthodontic standards. *Br Dent J* 1983; **155**: 133–5.

55. Sims-Williams J H, Brown I D, Matthewman A, Stephens C D. A computer controlled expert system for orthodontic advice. *Br Dent J* 1987; **163**: 161–9.

56. Appropriate Health Resources and Technologies Action Group Ltd. *Assisting dental education and dental health in developing countries.* A symposium. London: AHRTAG, 1981.

57. Bohannan H M. The impact of decreasing caries prevalence: implications for dental education. *J Dent Res* 1982; **61**(Sp.iss): 1369–77.

58. Lester K S. The future of conservative dentistry. *Aust Dent J* 1986; **31**: 111–6.

59. Elderton R J, Dowell T B. Decisions in forward-looking oral health care: summary statement. *Br Dent J* 1989; **166**: 467–9.

Further reading

Bailit H L, Braun R, Maryniuk G A, Camp P. "Is periodontal disease the primary cause of tooth extraction in adults?" *JADA* 1987; **114**: 40–5.

Craig G G, Powell K R, Cooper M H. Caries progression in primary molars: 24-month results from a minimal treatment programme. *Comm Dent Oral Epidemiol* 1981; **9**: 260–5.

Elderton R J. Restorative dentistry: 2. Prospects for the future. *Dent Update* 1986; **13**: 161–4, 166–8.

Genco R J. Pathogenesis of periodontal disease: new concepts. *J Canad Dent Assn* 1984; **50**: 391–5.

Granath L, McHugh W D (eds). *Systematized prevention of oral disease: Theory and practice.* Boca Raton: CRC Press, 1986.

Griffiths G S G, Wilton J M A, Curtis M A et al. Detection of high-risk groups and individuals for periodontal diseases: Clinical assessment of the periodontium. *J Clin Perio* 1988; **15**: 403–10.

Johnson N W (ed). 1989. *Oral cancer: Detection of patients and lesions at risk.* Cambridge: Cambridge University Press, 1989.

Larmas M. Simple tests for caries susceptibility. *Int Dent J* 1985; **35**: 109–17.

McLain J B, Proffitt W R. Oral health status in the United States: prevalence of malocclusion. *J Dent Educ* 1985; **49**: 386–96.

Meiers J C, Jensen M E. Management of the questionable carious fissure: invasive vs noninvasive techniques. *JADA* 1984; **108**: 64–8.

Renson C E, Crielaers P J A, Ibikunle S A J et al. Changing patterns of oral health and implications for oral health manpower. *Int Dent J* 1985; **35**: 235–51.

Scully C, Porter S R. Orofacial manifestations of HIV infection. *Lancet* 1988; **i**: 976–7.

Sheiham A. The epidemiology, etiology, and public health aspects of periodontal disease. *In* Grant D A, Stern I B, Listgarten M A (eds). *Periodontics in the tradition of Gottlieb and Orban.* pp 216–51. St Louis: C.V. Mosby Co, 1988.

Spencer A J. Contribution of fluoride vehicles to change in caries severity in Australian adolescents. *Comm Dent Oral Epidemiol* 1986; **14**: 238–41.

Wilton J M A, Griffths G S, Curtis M A et al. Detection of high-risk groups and individuals for periodontal diseases: Systemic predisposition and markers of general health. *J Clin Perio* 1988; **15**: 339–46.